ADVANCED
TAEKWONDO
SPARRING
and
HAPKIDO
TECHNIQUES

By Adam Gibson

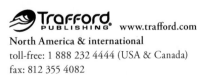 www.trafford.com
North America & international
toll-free: 1 888 232 4444 (USA & Canada)
fax: 812 355 4082

A Special Thanks

To my friends: Bob Cassidy, Jim Couch, Dave McFaul and Jill Hintz who volunteered their time to help me create this book. I would also like to thank my teacher Bill Wallace and his wife Kim Wallace who have been so supportive during some very uncomfortable times in my life. I could not have done this book without all of your support and kindness.

<u>Disclaimer</u>

Please note that the author and publisher of this book are NOT RESPONSIBLE in any manner whatsoever for any injury that may result from practicing the techniques and/or following the instructions given within. Since the physical activities described herein may be too strenuous in nature for some readers to engage in safely, it is essential that a physician be consulted prior to training.

Table of Contents

www.adamgibsontkd.com (For Updates on Videos and Books)

Introduction

I would like to warmly thank the reader for their interest in this book. This book was designed to give the beginner and black belt level martial artist a quick easy reference manual of how to deal with a large variation of different types of attacks that one may encounter in sparring or in a street situation. Most students when first beginning in a martial arts program are more interested in the actual defensive techniques than in kata (forms/patterns). Kata and/or traditional drills are usually based more on discipline rather than actual combat realism or knowledge. In much of the Kata practice today the students and even master level black belts don't even know what all the moves actually represent. Kata practice can be very important for development of good stances, footwork, concentration, focus, but still lacks the actual hands on practice necessary to develop good combat skills. Working with a partner is very important when developing your techniques. It allows you to test techniques in a controlled environment to see where you are weak and strong. It also allows you to see where your opponent is weak and strong. This book will give the martial artist a very strong base to improve one's defensive strategies but also start to learn how to develop techniques of their own. I hope all that read this book will gain knowledge that they could not find in other places. Good luck and have fun in your training.

Knowledge is Power,

Adam Gibson

Chapter One

Jab Defenses

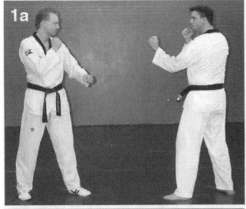

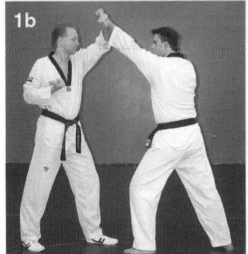

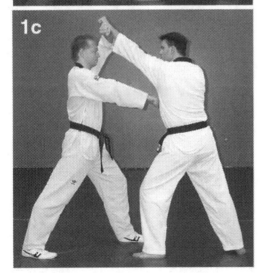

JAB DEFENSES (HIGH PUNCH)

TECHNIQUE #1

DEFENDER: RS ATTACKER: RS

1a) From solid fighting stance,
b) Lead high block,
c) and execute a reverse punch to the opponent's rib-cage while stepping into a forward walking stance(yell on the punch).

Note: Keep your back straight and remember to block first and then use your step forward to generate power for your punch.

4

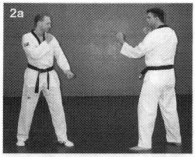

JAB DEFENSES (HIGH PUNCH)

TECHNIQUE #2

DEFENDER: RS   ATTACKER: RS

2a) From a solid fighting stance
b) Sidestep using your rear foot while simultaneously executing a knifehand block to the opponent's wrist,
c) Grab the opponent's wrist,
d) and execute a lead-leg roundhouse kick to the mid-section(yell on the kick).

Note: Strike with the instep of the foot.

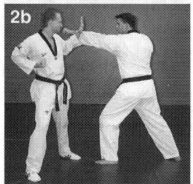

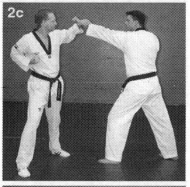

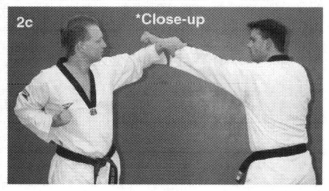

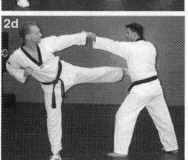

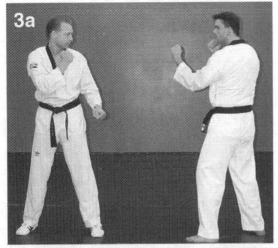

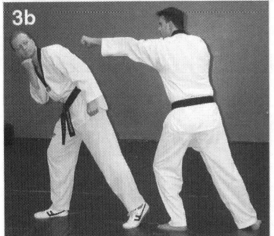

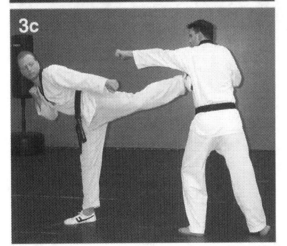

JAB DEFENSES (HIGH PUNCH)

TECHNIQUE #3

DEFENDER: RS   ATTACKER: RS

3a) From a solid fighting stance,
b) Lean your upper-body away from the punch,
c) and execute a lead leg side-kick to the opponent's rib cage(yell on the kick).

Note: Make sure to point your toes of your supporting foot in the opposite direction of your opponent. This will insure good stability and balance. If you do not point your toes in the opposite direction of the charging attacker you may roll over onto your ankle possibly breaking it, tearing some ligaments, or spraining it. Keep this in mind at all times.

6

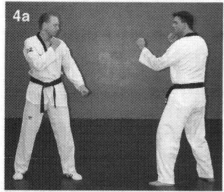

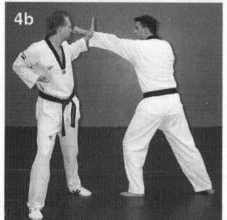

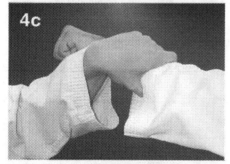

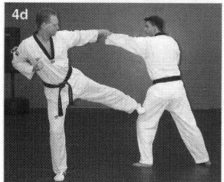

JAB DEFENSES (HIGH PUNCH)

TECHNIQUE #4

DEFENDER: RS   ATTACKER: RS

4a) From a solid fighting stance,
b) Sidestep with your rear foot while simultaneously executing a knifehand block to the opponent's wrist,
c) Grab your opponent's wrist,
d) and execute a lead leg sidekick to the opponent's forward knee(yell on the kick).

Note: This technique can be used to either break the knee or to take the opponent to the ground .

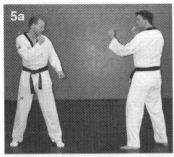

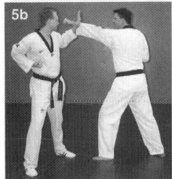

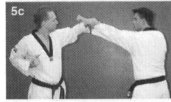

TECHNIQUE #5

5a) From a solid fighting stance,
b) Sidestep with your rear foot while simultaneously executing a knifehand block,
c) Grab the opponent's wrist,
d) Execute a (left hand) vertical punch to the rib-cage(to soften them up),
e) With your left foot step across to the right placing your buttocks against your opponent's hip area while raising their arm above your head,
f) and break the opponent's arm on your left shoulder holding on to their wrist with both your hands(yell on the break).
Note: Make sure your opponent's palm is facing the ceiling when you execute the arm-break.

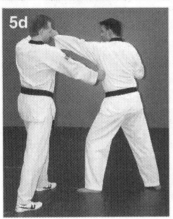

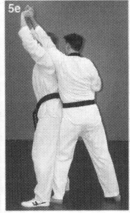

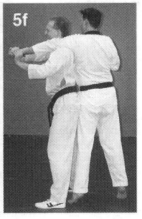

Chapter Two

Reverse Punch Defenses

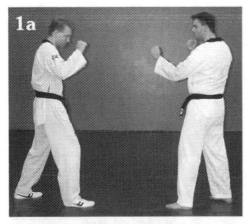

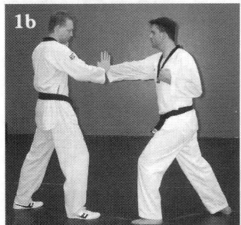

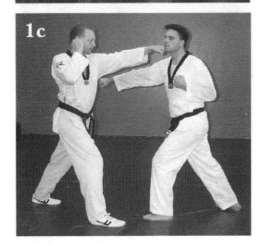

REVERSE PUNCH DEFENSES

TECHNIQUE #1

STANCE: Open-Stance

1a) From a solid fighting stance,
b) Execute a lead-palm block to the opponent's wrist,
c) and then execute a reverse punch to the opponent's face while stepping into a walking stance for power (yell on the punch).

Note: Make sure that the opponent's punch has cleared your body before you step in to execute the reverse punch to the opponent's face.

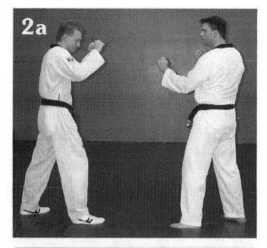

REVERSE PUNCH DEFENSES

TECHNIQUE #2

STANCE: Open-Stance

2a) From a solid fighting stance,
b) execute a rear palm block down to the opponent's wrist (twisting your upper body),
c) and simultaneously step forward with your rear foot and execute a reverse palm-heel strike to the opponent's nose(yell on strike).

Note: Think of the twisting action of the hips before the reverse palm-heel strike as similar to that of throwing a shot-put.

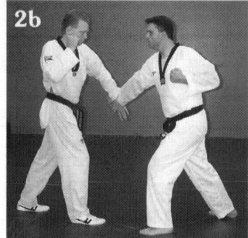

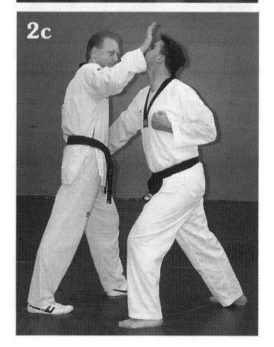

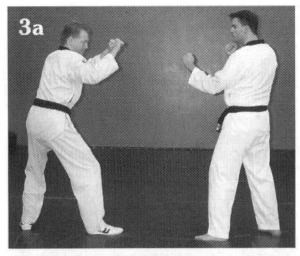

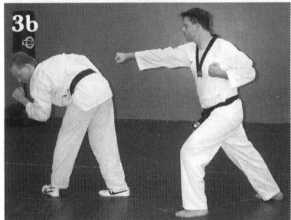

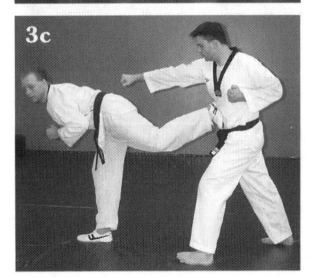

REVERSE PUNCH DEFENSES

TECHNIQUE #3

STANCE: Open-Stance

3a) From a solid fighting stance,
b) pivot your front foot so that your toes are pointing in the opposite direction of your opponent while simultaneously leaning out of range of your opponent's reverse punch,
c) and execute a turn back kick to the opponent's mid-section (yell on the kick).

Note: In order to keep from getting punched as you counter your opponent keep your back parallel to the floor. This way the punch will go over your back instead of into it.

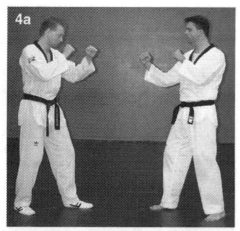

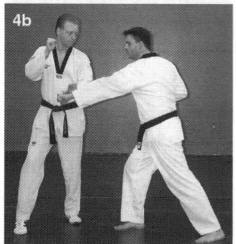

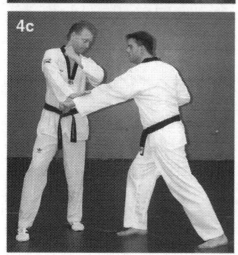

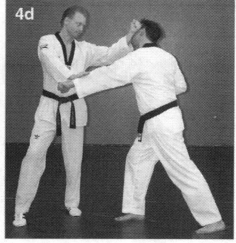

REVERSE PUNCH DEFENSES

TECHNIQUE #4

STANCE: Open-Stance

4a) From a solid fighting stance,
b) execute a lead palm block downwards while simultaneously pivoting 90-degrees on the balls of your feet,
c) Trap the opponent's wrist with your rear-hand(palm-down),
d) and execute a lead back-fist to the opponent's head (yell on strike).

Note: When you start in your fighting stance your body is facing almost square to your opponent. Then as they attack you pivot on the balls of your feet turning your body sideways taking the target away and off the straight line of attack. Your weight shifts to your forward leg as you strike to increase power.

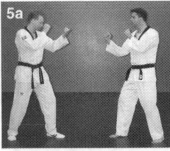

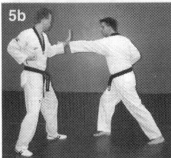

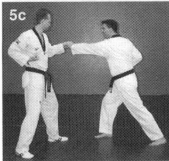

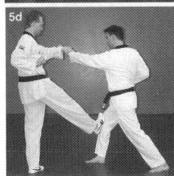

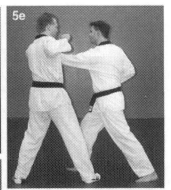

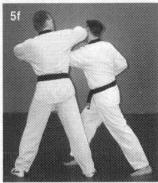

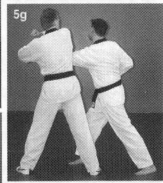

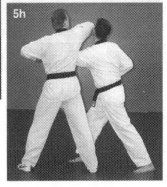

REVERSE PUNCH DEFENSES

TECHNIQUE #5

STANCE: Open-Stance

5a) From a solid fighting stance,
b) Sidestep with your rear foot while simultaneously executing a knife-hand block to the opponent's wrist,
c) grab the opponent's wrist,
d) execute a rear-leg front kick to the opponent's forward knee,
e) step down in between the opponent's feet,
f) execute a lead roundhouse elbow strike to the side of the opponent's head,
g-h) and then execute a lead jabbing elbow strike to the opponent's head (yell on the strike).

Note: Make sure that you do not let go of your opponent's wrist while executing the elbow strikes or they will be able to escape or punch you with their other hand.

Chapter Three

Hook Punch Defenses

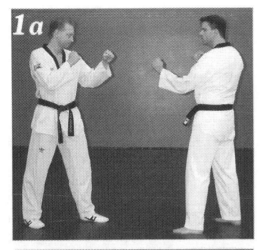

TECHNIQUE #1

STANCE: Closed-Stance

1a) From a solid fighting stance,
b) Execute a lead inside-outside forearm block to inside of the opponent's forearm,
c) and execute a reverse punch to nose (yell on the punch).

Note: Make sure that you do not block the opponent's punch at the elbow or their hook-punch will wrap around your block and hit you in the head as they intended. Try blocking between the middle of the forearm and the wrist to keep safe.

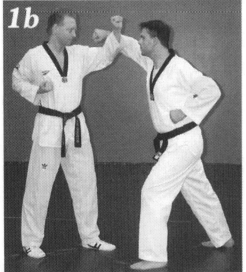

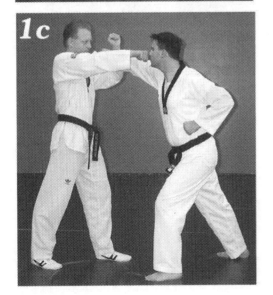

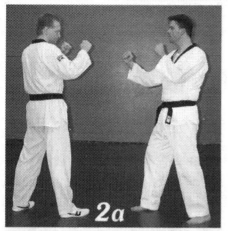

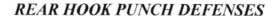
REAR HOOK PUNCH DEFENSES

TECHNIQUE #2

STANCE: Closed-Stance

2a) From a solid fighting stance,
b) Execute a lead inside-outside forearm block to opponents forearm,
c) Grab your opponent's bicep with your lead hand while simultaneously reaching behind the opponent's neck grabbing a nerve point with your fingers,
d) Pull your opponent towards you and execute an upward knee strike to the groin (yell on the strike).

Note: If your opponent is much taller than you striking to the groin is much easier and more effective than striking to the mid-section. If your opponent is big and strong you may not be able to get him bend over enough to get a clean knee-strike to the mid-section.

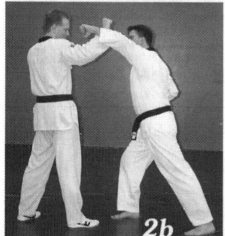

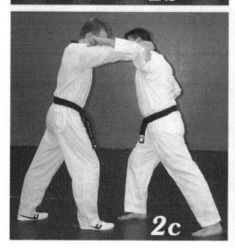

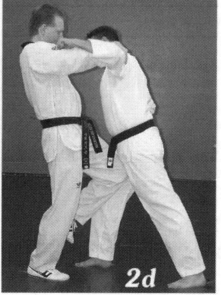

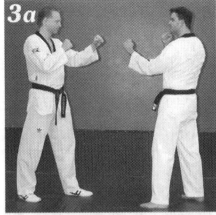

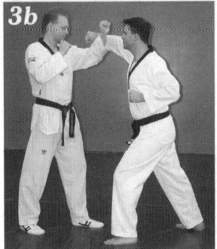

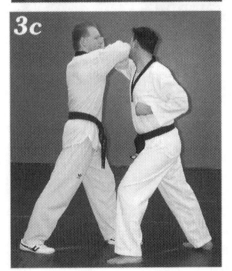

TECHNIQUE #3

STANCE: Closed-Stance

3a) From a solid fighting stance,
b) Execute a lead inside-outside forearm block to your opponent's forearm,
c) Step forward with your front foot and execute a reverse roundhouse elbow-strike to the side of the opponent's head (yell on the strike).

Note: To generate more power from your elbow strike twist your upper body into the strike while raising the heel of your rear foot. By raising the heel of your rear foot it will allow your knee to rotate inward which in turn will allow the maximum release of the hip. Hip release is the key to true power in all types of striking.

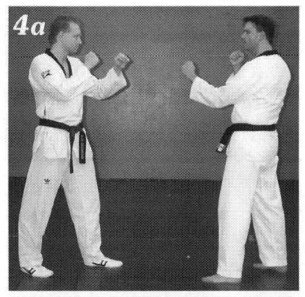

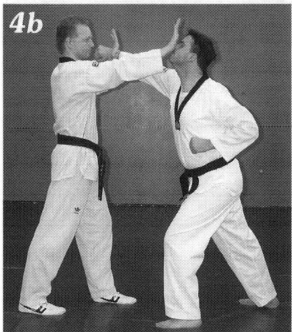

TECHNIQUE #4

STANCE: Closed-Stance

4a) From a solid fighting stance,
b) Simultaneously execute a lead knifehand block to the opponent's wrist and a reverse palm-heel strike to the opponent's nose (yell on the strike).

Note: Simultaneous blocking and striking techniques are very advanced and much practice is needed for effectiveness in real combat. Although after a level mastery has been attained they can be extremely lethal and end a fight very quickly.

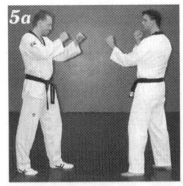

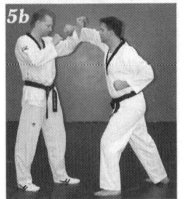

REAR HOOK PUNCH DEFENSES

TECHNIQUE #5

STANCE: Closed-Stance

5a) From a solid fighting stance,
b) Execute an inside-outside forearm block to opponent's forearm,
c-e) and execute a rear upper-cut to the opponent's mid-section (yell on the punch).

Note: When executing an upper-cut you must drive your fist upward in a scooping action with your arm. Notice in the below picture(5e) the opponent is almost being lifted off the floor in an upward fashion. This demonstrates the upward scooping motion of the upper-cut punch.

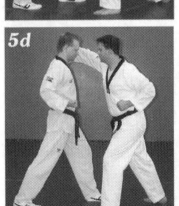

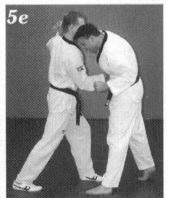

Chapter Four

Backfist Defenses

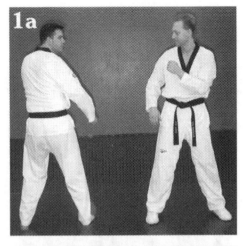

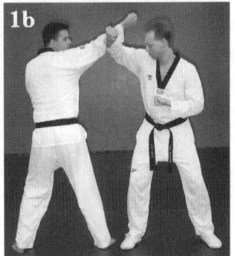

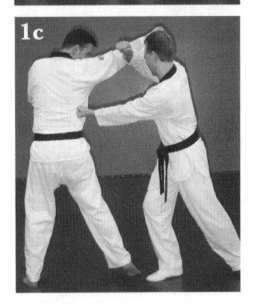

BACKFIST DEFENSES

TECHNIQUE #1

STANCE: Closed-Stance

1a) From a solid fighting stance,
b) Execute a high block with your forward arm,
c) and execute an under-cut punch to rib-cage (yell on the punch).

Note: Remember that the under-cut punch is a straight-line technique. It is different than an upper-cut punch. An upper-cut punch is an arcing/scooping action and the under-cut punch once again travels in a straight line only.

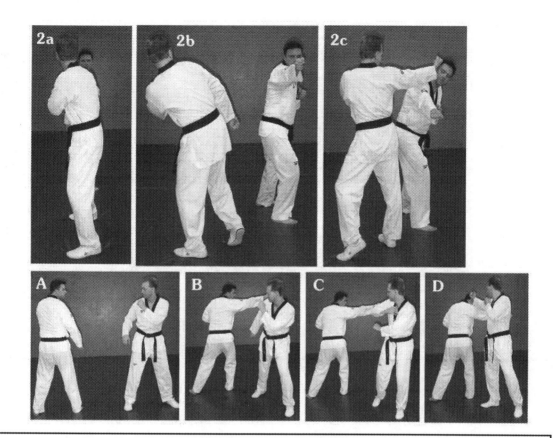

BACKFIST DEFENSES

TECHNIQUE #2

STANCE: Closed-Stance

2a) From solid fighting stance,
b) Sidestep with your rear foot while deaking your head out of range of the opponent's backfist,
c) and execute a lead backfist to the opponent's head (yell on the backfist).

Note: When you sidestep as in the above picture 2b) your body weight shifts to your rear foot to allow you to lean out of your opponent's striking range. Then when you are safely out of range you push off of your rear-foot, which is like a coiled-spring because your knee is slightly bent, and execute the backfist transferring your body weight to your front foot as seen in picture 2c. Weight transfer from rear to front foot is the key to power and speed in the above technique.

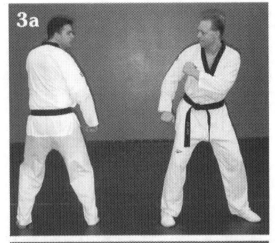

BACKFIST DEFENSES

TECHNIQUE #3

STANCE: Closed-Stance

3a) From a solid fighting stance,
b) Lean back out of range of the punch while simultaneously pointing your toes in the opposite direction of your incoming opponent,
c) and execute a lead leg stopping side-kick to rib cage (yell on the kick).

Note: The body lean as seen in picture 3b is very crucial in the success of this technique. If your body is too upright you risk getting hit. You goal is to take the target away from your opponent while making your opponent open up their rib-cage for your counter-attack.

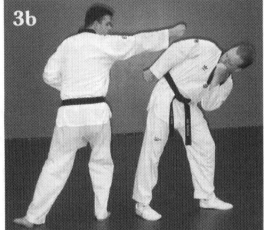

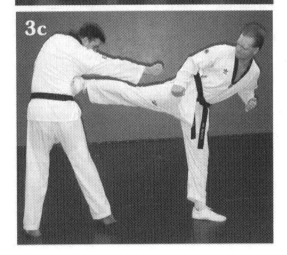

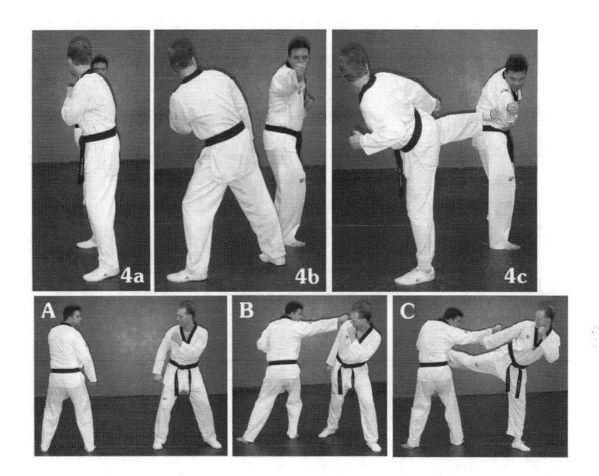

TECHNIQUE #4

STANCE: Closed-Stance

4a) From a solid fighting stance,
b) Sidestep with your rear foot out of range of your opponent's backfist,
c) and execute a lead leg roundhouse kick to the opponent's mid-section (yell on the kick).

Note: Make sure that when you sidestep as in the above picture 4b) that you lean your head out of range so that you are out of your opponent's striking range.

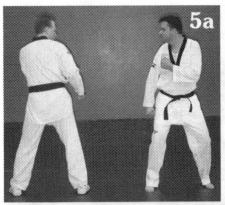 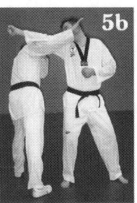

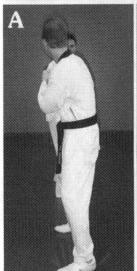 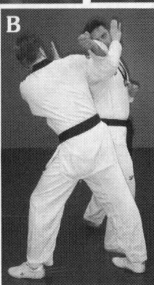 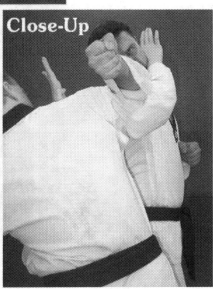

TECHNIQUE #5

STANCE: Closed-Stance

5a) From a solid fighting stance,
b) Sidestep with your rear foot while simultaneously executing a lead ridgehand strike to the opponent's head (yell on the ridgehand strike).

Note: Use a rear open-hand for protection on the lead side of your face. In other words protect the side of your face which is closest to your opponent.

Chapter Five

Front Kick Defenses

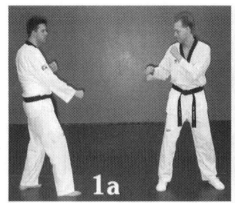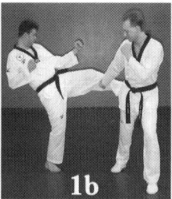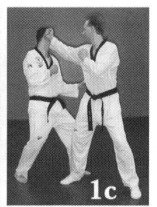

FRONT SNAP KICK DEFENSES

TECHNIQUE #1

STANCE: Closed-Stance

1a) From a solid fighting stance,

b) Side step with your rear foot while simultaneously executing a closed-fisted low block with your lead arm,

c) and execute a lead backfist to the opponent's head (yell on the backfist).

Note: When executing sidestepping techniques as in the above be sure not to make your stance too wide. If your stance is too wide it is difficult to move and react quickly. Fighting in a traditional riding-horse stance is not recommended. A riding-horse stance is generally two shoulder-widths wide or more. Your fighting stance should be a shoulder-width or one and a half shoulder-widths wide maximum.

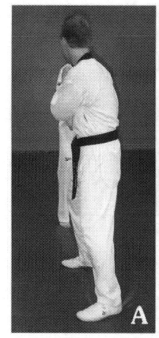 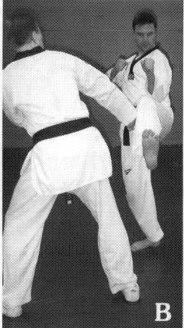 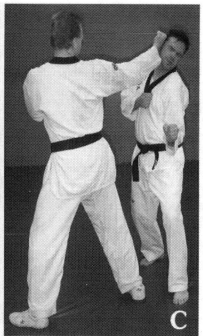

TECHNIQUE #1(REAR-VIEW)

STANCE: Closed-Stance

Note: When executing the low block as is in the above picture B) make sure you block between the knee and ankle of the opponent for best results. Also if you find that you are too far away from your opponent after you block push hard off of your rear foot and step forward with your lead foot and execute the backfist to the head as in picture C). Pushing off of your rear foot will put your body weight behind your counter backfist resulting in increased power.

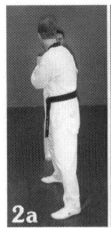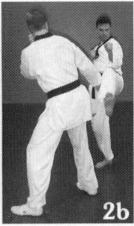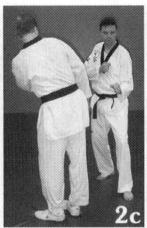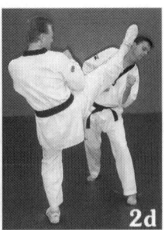

FRONT SNAP KICK DEFENSES

TECHNIQUE #2

STANCE: Closed-Stance

2a) From a solid fighting stance,

b) Side step with your rear foot and simultaneously execute a closed-fisted low block,

c) Slide your rear foot up to your front foot,

d) and execute a lead leg crescent kick to the opponent's face (strike with the side of your instep and yell on the kick).

Note: When side stepping be sure to lean away as in picture 2b) to avoid being hit.

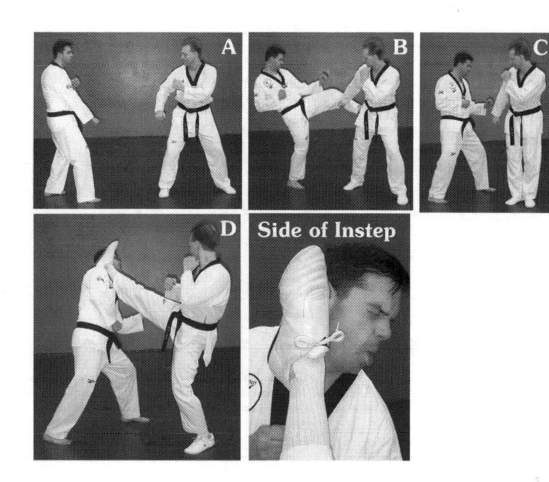

FRONT SNAP KICK DEFENSES

TECHNIQUE #2(SIDE-VIEW)

STANCE: Closed-Stance

Note: When striking with the crescent kick utilize the side of the instep or sometimes called the blade of the foot.

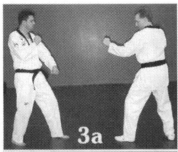
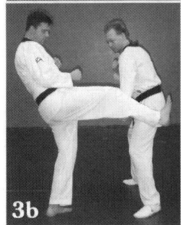
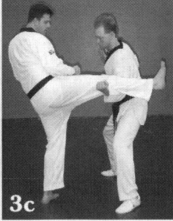
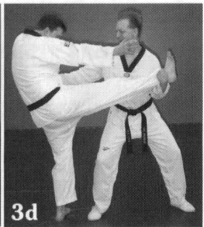

FRONT SNAP KICK DEFENSES

TECHNIQUE #3

STANCE: Closed-Stance

3a) From a solid fighting stance,
b) Sidestep with your rear foot and execute a closed-fisted low block,
c) Continue through with the low-block and hook your lead forearm under the ankle or calf of the opponent,
d) With your rear foot step forward between your opponent's legs execute a palm-heel strike to the opponent's mid-section knocking the opponent to the ground (yell on the palm-heel strike).

Note: The deeper you step in between your opponent's legs the more power you will generate from your strike therefore increasing the ability to take your opponent completely of their feet.

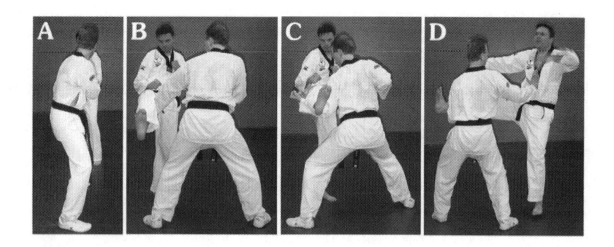

FRONT SNAP KICK DEFENSES

TECHNIQUE #3(REAR-VIEW)

STANCE: Closed-Stance

Note: Make sure you keep your fingers kept in a closed fist position when hooking your opponent's kicking leg. This is to avoid getting them broken if you misjudge or mistime your block.

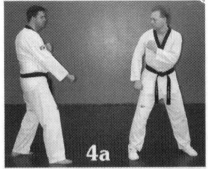

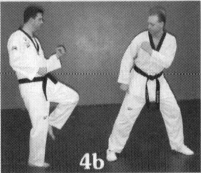

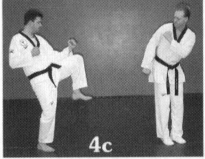

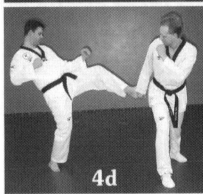

FRONT SNAP KICK DEFENSES

TECHNIQUE #4

STANCE: Closed-Stance

4a) From a solid fighting stance,
b) Step back with your rear foot about 10 inches,
c) Then slide your lead foot to your rear foot,
d) Then sidestep with your lead foot out to the same side as your stomach,
e) Draw your rear foot behind your lead foot,
f) and execute a lead leg hook-kick to the opponent's head (yell on the kick).

Note: Lateral footwork is the most difficult to master. The above technique must be practiced over and over and over again to develop proficiency in sparring.

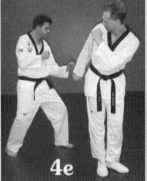

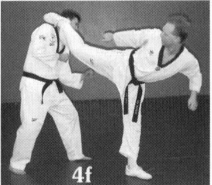

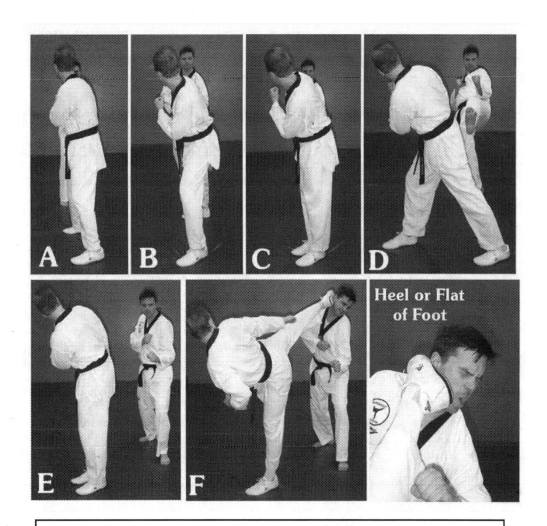

Heel or Flat of Foot

FRONT SNAP KICK DEFENSES

TECHNIQUE #4(REAR-VIEW)

STANCE: Closed-Stance

Note: When using the hook kick strike with the heel for power and use the bottom or flat of the foot for reach.

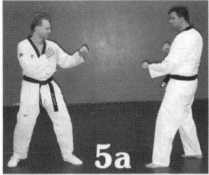

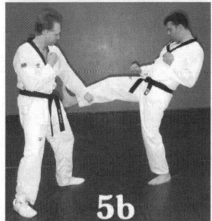

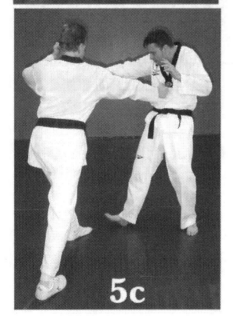

FRONT SNAP KICK DEFENSES

TECHNIQUE #5

STANCE: Closed-Stance

5a) From a solid fighting stance,
b) Side step with your rear foot and simultaneously execute a close-fisted low block to the opponent's kicking leg,
c) and execute a rear vertical punch to the opponent's mid-section (yell on the punch).

Note: In a real situation it is most beneficial to strike the opponent just before their kicking foot hits the floor. This will prevent the opponent from a follow-up technique plus catch them off balance possibly knocking them to the ground.

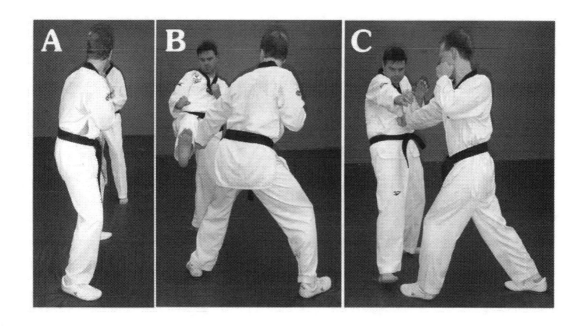

FRONT SNAP KICK DEFENSES

TECHNIQUE #5(REAR-VIEW)

STANCE: Closed-Stance

Note: For increased power in your punch twist your hips until your upper-body is perpendicular to your opponent's mid-section as seen in the above picture C).

Chapter Six

Roundhouse Kick Defenses

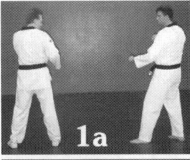

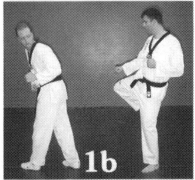

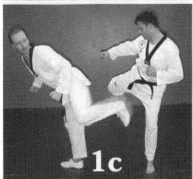

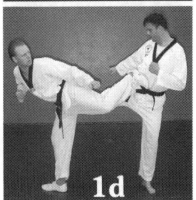

ROUNDHOUSE KICK DEFENSES

TECHNIQUE #1

STANCE: Open-Stance

1a) From a solid fighting stance,
b-d) and execute a turn back kick to the
opponent's mid-section before they can
complete their kick(yell on the kick).

*Note: In order to have a lightning fast
counter turn back kick your fighting
stance should not be anymore than a
shoulder-width apart. The wider your
stance, the more distance your foot has to
travel to the target.*

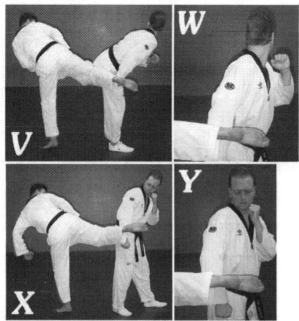

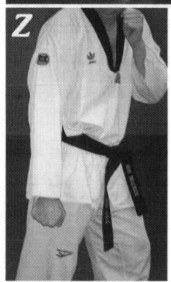

ROUNDHOUSE KICK DEFENSES

TECHNIQUE #1
"Important-TIP"

STANCE: Open-Stance

Note: When executing a counter turn back kick it is very important to protect your rib-cage with your lead forearm. The reason for this is because if you don't beat your opponent to the kick your rib-cage will be open to be scored on. The advantage of having your lead forearm in front of your rib-cage is not only to prevent you from getting your ribs broken, but you can use it to block and still finish your counter attack.

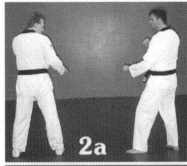

2a

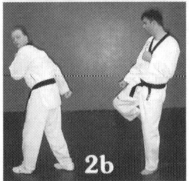

2b

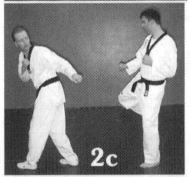

2c

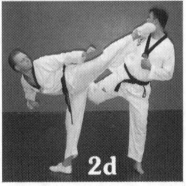

2d

ROUNDHOUSE KICK DEFENSES

TECHNIQUE #2

STANCE: Open-Stance

2a) From a solid fighting stance,
b-d) execute a spinning hook kick to the opponent's head as they attack(yell on the kick).

Note: As soon as you see the opponent's forward movement (their hips and shoulders turning) it is time to release your counter spinning hook kick.

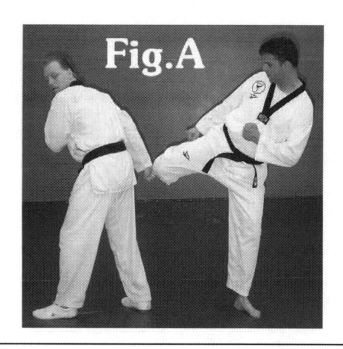

Fig.A

ROUNDHOUSE KICK DEFENSES

TECHNIQUE #2
"Important Tip"

STANCE: Open-Stance

Note: Just as in technique #1 the placement of the forearm is very important for defensive purposes. The spinning hook kick counter attack is identical to that of the turn back kick counter attack other than the fact that you are kicking the opponent in the head instead of the body. The defensive body posturing is exactly the same.

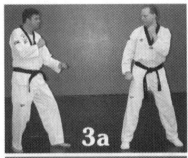

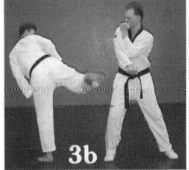

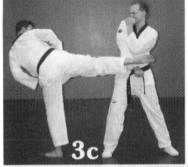

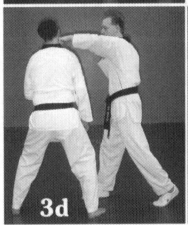

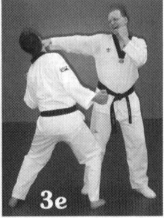

TECHNIQUE #3

STANCE: Open-Stance

3a) From a solid fighting stance,
b-c) Execute a low-high forearm block,
d) Execute a reverse punch to the opponent's head,
e) and execute a jab punch to the opponent's head (yell on the punch).

Note: This technique is excellent to use when you do not have time to get out of the way of the opponent's kick.

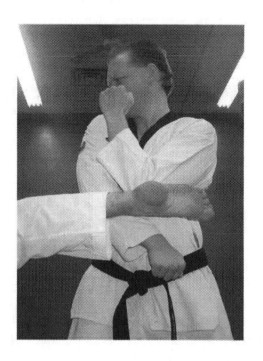

ROUNDHOUSE KICK DEFENSES

TECHNIQUE #3 (CLOSE-UP)

STANCE: Open-Stance

Note: It is very important to make sure that your elbows touch when blocking your opponent's kick. The rear hand protects your jaw, your elbows protect your solar-plexus, and your lead forearm and hand protects your stomach and groin.

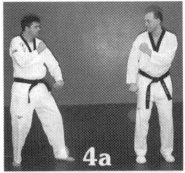

4a

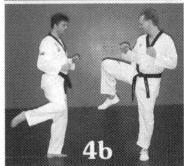

4b

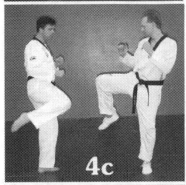

4c

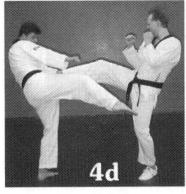

4d

ROUNDHOUSE KICK DEFENSES

TECHNIQUE #4

STANCE: Open-Stance

4a) From a solid fighting stance,
b-d) Execute a lead leg front kick to the opponent's body as they attempt to attack(yell on the kick).

Note: In order to utilize the stopping front kick effectively you must start in a "defensive fighting stance". The "defensive fighting stance" is no more than a shoulder-width wide. Using a stance that is only a shoulder-width wide will allow you to use your lead-leg faster than from a wider stance. From a "defensive fighting stance" all you have to do is lift your knee and kick. The supporting leg is also much closer to your opponent when using a shorter stance. A shorter stance eliminates the necessity of having to slide your rear foot up to your front foot to get close enough to intercept your opponent's kick.

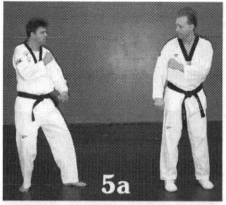

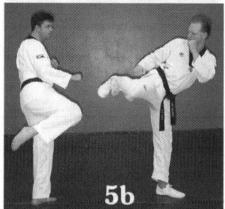

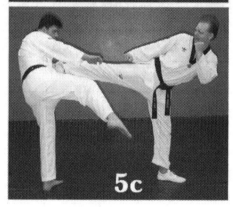

ROUNDHOUSE KICK DEFENSES

TECHNIQUE #5

STANCE: Open-Stance

5a) From a solid fighting stance,
b-c) Execute a lead leg stopping side-kick to the opponent's mid-section as they attempt to attack(yell on the kick).

Note: In order to utilize the stopping sidekick effectively you must start in a "defensive fighting stance". The "defensive fighting stance" is no more than a shoulder-width wide. Using a stance that is only a shoulder-width wide will allow you to use your lead-leg faster than from a wider stance. From a "defensive fighting stance" all you have to do is lift your knee and kick. The supporting leg is also much closer to your opponent when using a shorter stance. A shorter stance eliminates the necessity of having to slide your rear foot up to your front foot to get close enough to intercept your opponent's kick.

Chapter Seven

Sidekick Defenses

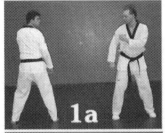

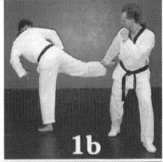

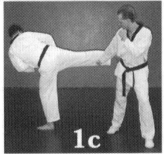

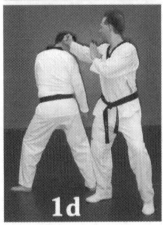

SIDEKICK DEFENSES

TECHNIQUE #1

STANCE: Closed-Stance

1a) From a solid fighting stance,
b-c) Side step with your rear foot to avoid being hit by your opponent's sidekick while simultaneously executing a lead low block to the opponent's calf/ankle area,
d) and execute a back-fist to the opponent's head (yell on the strike).

Note: Make sure you shift your body weight to your rear foot as you sidestep. This will enable you to lean your upper body out of range of your opponent's sidekick.

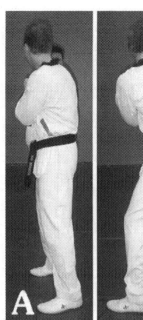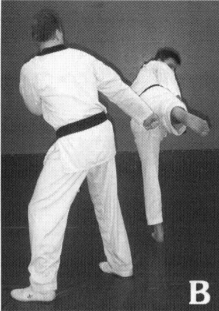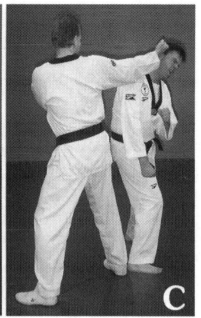

SIDEKICK DEFENSES

TECHNIQUE #1(REAR-VIEW)

STANCE: Closed-Stance

Note: If you wind up too far away from your opponent after you sidestep and block, push hard off of your rear foot and step forward with your lead foot to get back into range to execute the backfist. You will also find that this will give added power in your strike.

51

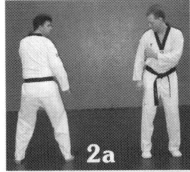

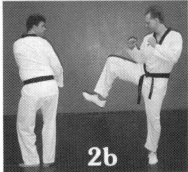

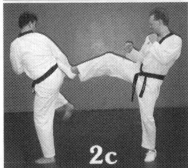

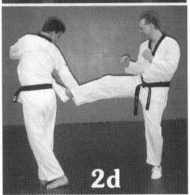

TECHNIQUE #2

STANCE: Closed-Stance

2a) From a solid fighting stance,
b-d) Execute a lead leg front kick to the opponent's rib-cage/hip area (yell on the kick).

Note: Make sure you start from a "defensive fighting stance" as explained in the "Roundhouse Kick Defenses" section of this book. Your fighting stance should only be one shoulder-width apart. The second key to effectively using this technique is to catch your opponent on his approaching footwork. In this example the attacker is countered as he slides his leg up to the cover distance necessary to reach the defender. The attacker is completely neutralized before he has the opportunity to finish his attack.

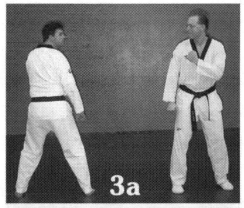

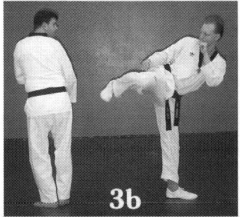

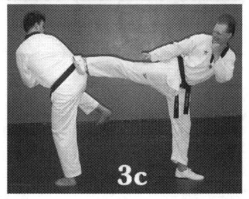

SIDEKICK DEFENSES

TECHNIQUE #3

STANCE: Closed-Stance

3a) From a solid fighting stance,
b) Execute a stopping sidekick to the opponent's rib-cage/hip area (yell on the kick).

Note: Make sure you start from a "defensive fighting stance" as explained in the "Roundhouse Kick Defenses" section of this book. Your fighting stance should only be one shoulder-width apart. The second key to effectively using this technique is to catch your opponent on his approaching footwork. In this example the attacker is countered as he slides his leg up to the cover distance necessary to reach the defender. The attacker is completely neutralized before he has the opportunity to finish his attack.

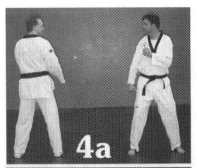

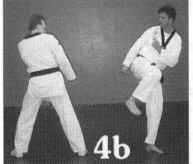

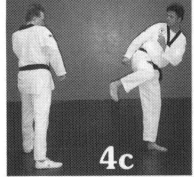

SIDEKICK DEFENSES

TECHNIQUE #4

STANCE: Closed-Stance

4a) From a solid fighting stance,
b) Step back with your rear foot,
c) Draw your lead foot 45 degrees backwards off the line of fire,
d) Draw your rear foot behind your lead foot,
e) and execute a lead leg roundhouse kick to the opponent's head (yell on the kick).

Note: This technique will greatly help the martial artist in developing advanced defensive footwork. Split second timing is required for this type of maneuver.

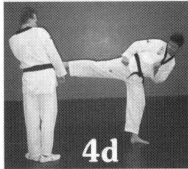

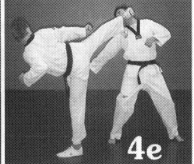

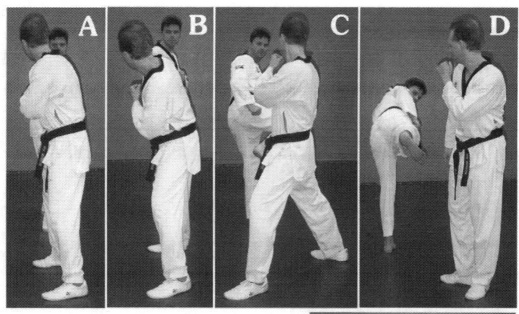

SIDEKICK DEFENSES

TECHNIQUE #4
REAR-VIEW

STANCE: Closed-Stance

Note: Lateral footwork techniques can be difficult to master, but when that mastery comes you will become extremely deceptive during sparring. The opponent who hardly ever gets hit is usually the one who's always left standing.

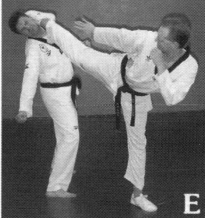

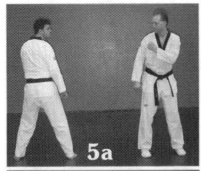

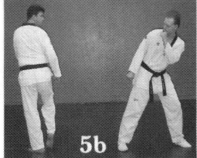

SIDEKICK DEFENSES

TECHNIQUE #5

STANCE: Closed-Stance

5a) From a solid fighting stance,

b) Step back with your rear foot,

c) Draw your lead foot to your rear foot,

d) Sidestep off the "line of fire" to the same side as your belly,

e) Draw your rear foot to your lead foot,

f) and execute a lead leg hook-kick to the opponent's head (yell on the kick).

Note: Once again this is another piece of lateral footwork which must be practiced over and over again to become second nature during sparring.

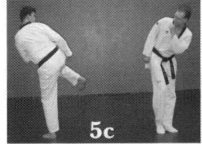

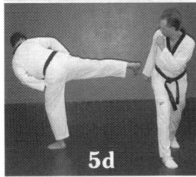

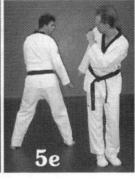

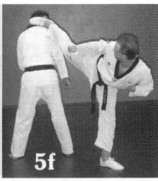

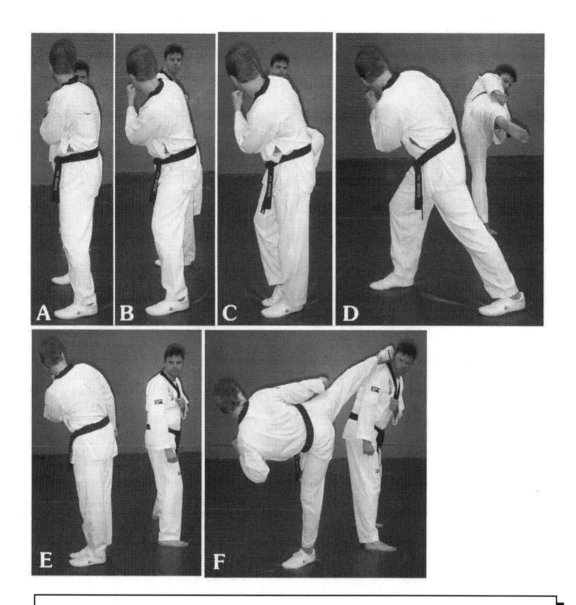

SIDEKICK DEFENSES

TECHNIQUE #5(REAR-VIEW)

STANCE: Closed-Stance

Note: When you sidestep be sure to lean your upper body away from the opponent's attack as in the above pictures.

Chapter Eight

Turn Back Kick Defenses

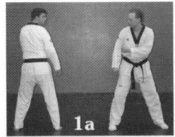

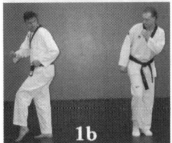

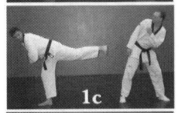

TURN BACK KICK DEFENSES

TECHNIQUE #1

STANCE: Closed-Stance

1a) From a solid fighting stance,
b-c) Skip back out of range of the opponent's turn back kick,
d) and execute a rear leg roundhouse kick to the opponent's mid-section,
e) retract your leg back to chamber-position,
f) and execute a roundhouse kick to the opponent's head (yell on the kick).

Note: Try practicing this technique in a fighting stance that is about two shoulder-widths wide. Some beginner students have difficulties with the footwork if they start in a shorter fighting stances.

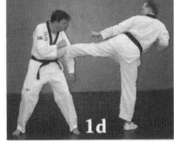

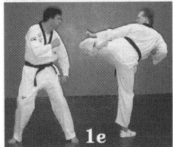

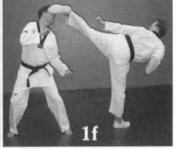

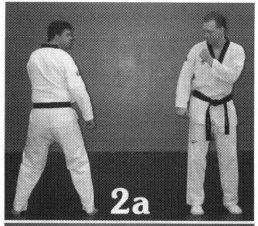

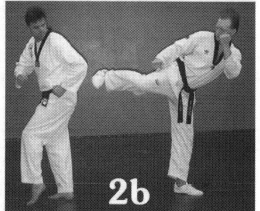

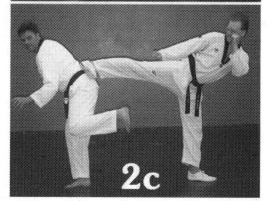

TURN BACK KICK DEFENSES

TECHNIQUE #2

STANCE: Closed-Stance

2a) From a solid fighting stance,
b-c) Execute a lead leg side-kick to the opponent's hip/kidney area as they attempt to attack(yell on the kick).

Note: Once again using the "defensive fighting stance" you keep your feet only one shoulder-width apart so that you can intercept your opponent with your sidekick before they can complete their turn back kick.

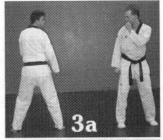

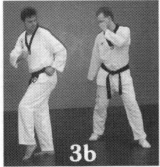

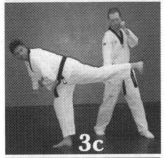

TURN BACK KICK DEFENSES

TECHNIQUE #3

STANCE: Closed-Stance

3a) From a solid fighting stance,
b-c) Sidestep with your lead foot towards the same side as your back while simultaneously executing a lead low forearm block to the opponent's kicking leg,
d) and execute a reverse punch to the opponent's head (yell on the punch).

Note: It is not important that your lead low forearm block actually make contact with your opponent's leg. It's there just incase your opponent's turn back kick arcs and follows you as you sidestep. It is always a good idea to have something between you and your opponent incase your footwork goes wrong.

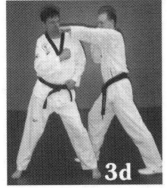

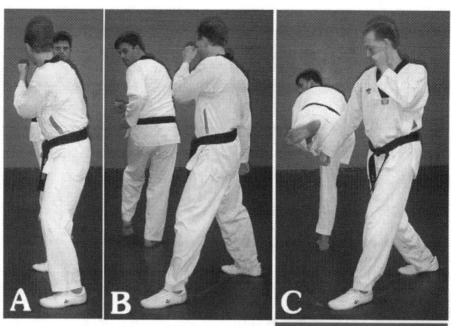

TURN BACK KICK DEFENSES

TECHNIQUE #3 (REAR-VIEW)

STANCE: Closed-Stance

Note: The key to this technique is to get off the turn back kick's trajectory or "line of fire". In the beginning this piece of lateral footwork will feel a little awkward to the beginner, but will eventually become easier after hours of repetition have been endured.

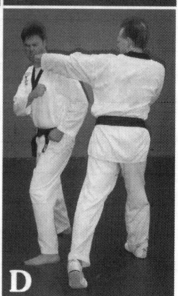

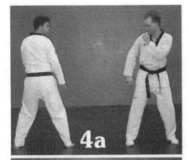

4a

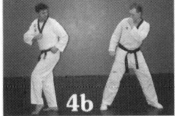

4b

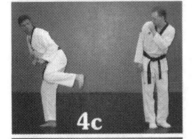

4c

TURN BACK KICK DEFENSES

TECHNIQUE #4

STANCE: Closed-Stance

4a) From a solid fighting stance,
b) Step back with your rear foot,
c) Pull your front foot to your rear foot,
d-e) Step with your front foot to the same side as your stomach,
f) Draw your rear foot behind your front foot,
g) and execute a lead leg hook-kick to the head (yell on the kick).

Note: For best results you must be out of your opponent's kicking range and ready to counter either just before their kicking foot hits the floor or just as it touches the floor. Always remember that your opponent is the most dangerous when he has both feet on the ground and is balanced. If you can catch him while he is on one foot or is trying to regain his balance you have the upper hand.

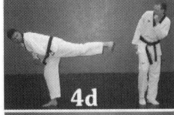

4d

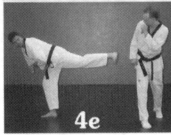

4e

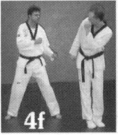

4f

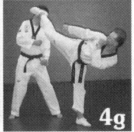

4g

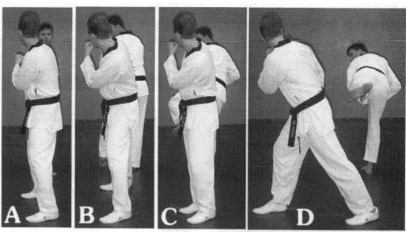

TURN BACK KICK DEFENSES

TECHNIQUE #4

STANCE: Closed-Stance

Note: Once again as seen in picture D) on this page the body lean defense is implemented to help avoid your opponent's attack. Learning how to avoid your opponent's offensive movements through footwork and body positioning (eg. Body-leaning) is the true path to becoming a master of defensive fighting.

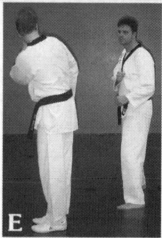

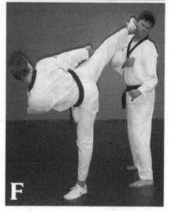

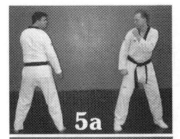

5a

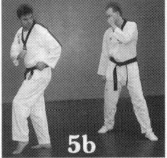

5b

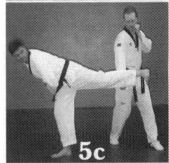

5c

TURN BACK KICK DEFENSES

TECHNIQUE #5

STANCE: Closed-Stance

5a) From a solid fighting stance,
b) sidestep with your lead foot to the same side as
your back while keeping your lead forearm low
in front of your rib-cage,
c) turn your upper body towards your opponent
executing a low forearm block to your opponent's
kicking leg,
d) trap you're your opponent's lead arm at their
triceps with a rear open palm,
e) and execute a lead backfist (right) to the head
(yell on the backfist).

*Note: For extra power on your backfist transfer
your body weight to your lead foot as you strike.*

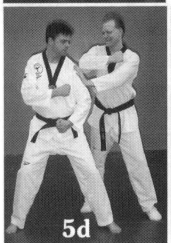

5d

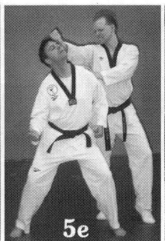

5e

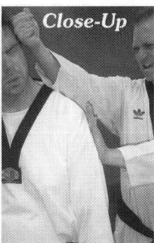

Close-Up

66

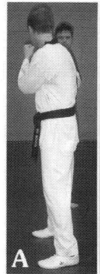
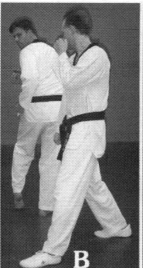
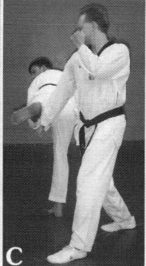
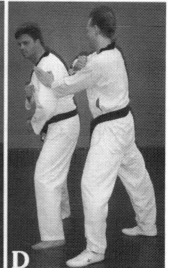

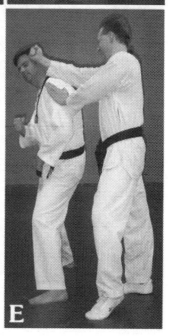

TURN BACK KICK DEFENSES

TECHNIQUE #5

STANCE: Closed-Stance

Note: The position of your lead forearm is very important when utilizing this technique. It is used to help protect your rib-cage, stomach and groin. An improper calculation can allow your opponent's turn back kick to score. The footwork utilized for this technique will feel slightly awkward in the beginning, but in time will become easier with constant practice.

Chapter Nine

Straight Wrist-Grab Defenses

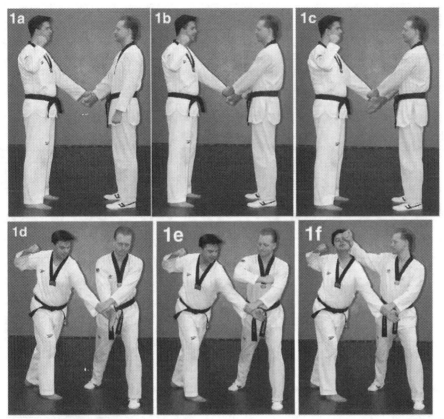

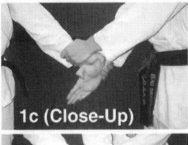

1c (Close-Up)

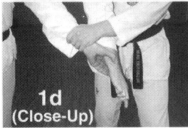

1d (Close-Up)

HAPKIDO:
STRAIGHT WRIST GRAB

TECHNIQUE #1

1a) The opponent grabs your wrist,
b) Grab their wrist with your opposite hand,
c-d) Step into a walking stance while simultaneously pulling the opponent with you to get them off balance and twisting your palm down and towards you to escape their grip,
e-f) and execute a lead backfist to the opponent's head (yell on the strike).

Note: Examine pictures 1c(Close-Up) and 1d(Close-Up) study the mechanics of escaping your opponent's grip. The key is to break out at the opponent's thumb. The thumb is the weak point in your opponent's grip.

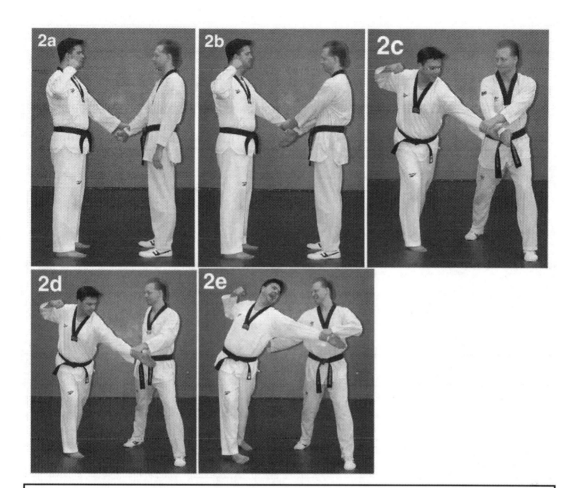

HAPKIDO:
STRAIGHT WRIST GRAB

TECHNIQUE #2

1a) The opponent grabs your wrist,
b) Grab their wrist with your opposite hand,
c) Step into a walking stance while simultaneously pulling the opponent with you to get them off balance and twisting your palm down and towards you to escape their grip,
d) Pull your fist to chamber position just above your hip,
e) and execute a lead vertical punch to the opponent's rib-cage (yell on the strike).

Note: Stepping to get your opponent off balance while simultaneously twisting your palm downwards will enhance your ability to escape the opponent's grip. The opponent is forced to deal with more than one task. He has to try to maintain his balance while trying to keep control of your wrist.

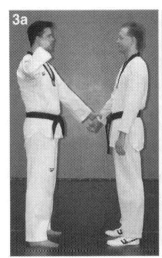

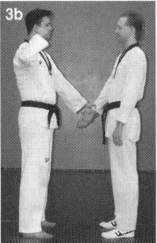

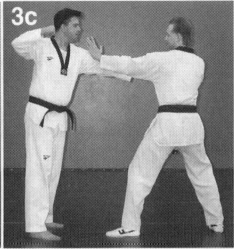

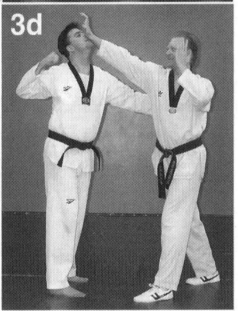

HAPKIDO:
STRAIGHT WRIST GRAB

TECHNIQUE #3

3a) The opponent grabs your wrist,
b) Extend your fingers out straight in a knifehand position,
c) Step back with the same foot that is on the same side as you're being grabbed (keep your lead guard up as your knifehand breaks out at the opponent's thumb),
d) and execute a reverse palm-heel strike to the opponent's nose (yell on the strike).

Note: If you wind up too far away from your opponent push off of your rear foot and step forward with your front foot to cover the distance.

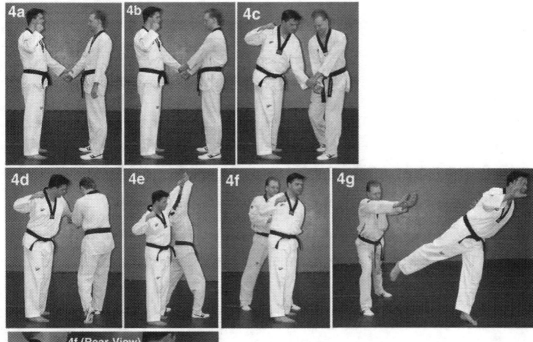

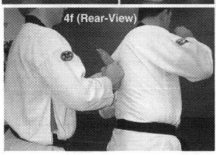

4f (Rear-View)

HAPKIDO:
STRAIGHT WRIST GRAB

TECHNIQUE #4

4a) The opponent grabs your wrist,
b) With your opposite hand grab your opponent's wrist,
c) Execute a body fake by tugging your opponent's arm on a 45-degree angle pulling the opponent off balance,
d-e) Step across while going underneath opponent's arm,
f-g) Put the opponent's arm behind their back and push with both hands, taking a full walking stance step forward (yell on the push forward to release the "ki" energy).

Note: When executing the body fake tug down on the opponent's arm on a 45-degree angle. Think of the opponent's wrist like a knot in the rope. The idea is to make the opponent's shoulder drop lower than their opposite shoulder.

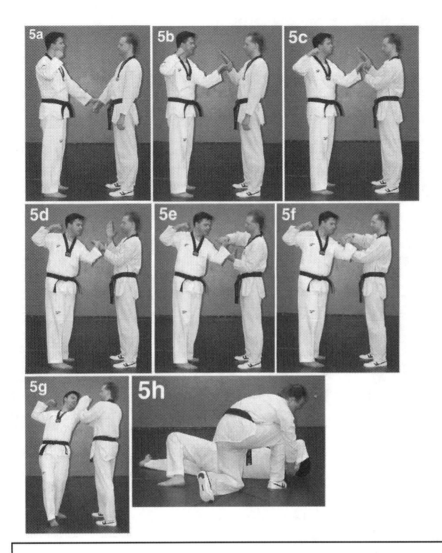

HAPKIDO:
STRAIGHT WRIST GRAB

TECHNIQUE #5

5a) The opponent grabs your wrist,
b-d) Rotate your palm upwards making your palm face you while your opposite hand implements a wrist lock position,
e-f) Your opposite hands slips out and comes back into reinforce a wrist-lock,
g) Tilt your opponent's elbow up towards the ceiling until their spine arches backwards,
h) Drop to the knee that's closest to your opponent, taking them to the ground (yell on the takedown).

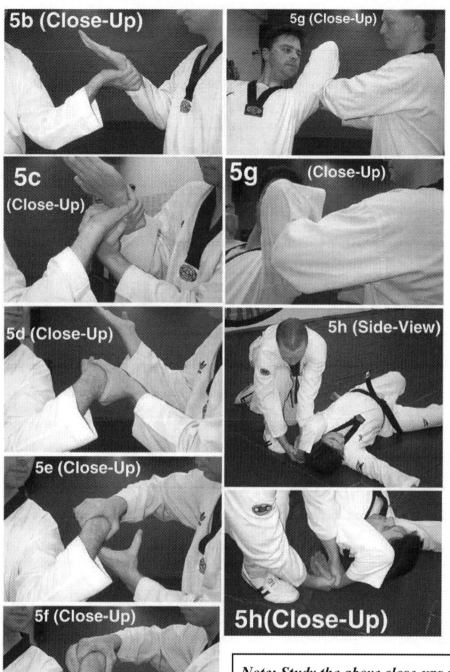

5b (Close-Up)

5g (Close-Up)

5c (Close-Up)

5g (Close-Up)

5d (Close-Up)

5h (Side-View)

5e (Close-Up)

5f (Close-Up)

5h (Close-Up)

Note: Study the above close-ups so that you can master the hand grips and changes that are required for this intricate wrist-lock technique. Practicing of this technique on a regular basis will help develop hand-speed and coordination.

Chapter Ten

Cross Wrist-Grab Defenses

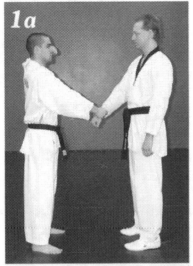

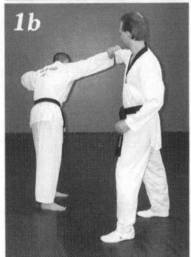

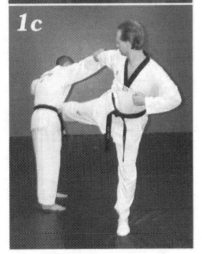

HAPKIDO:
CROSS WRIST GRAB

TECHNIQUE #1

1a) The opponent grabs your wrist,
b) Reverse the opponent's grab using a small clockwise circular movement (grabbing his wrist) while sidestepping with your opposite foot,
c) and execute lead leg roundhouse kick to the opponent's mid-section (yell on the kick).

Note: It is very important to sidestep far enough away from the opponent so that they can not reach you with their free hand.

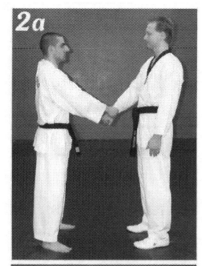

HAPKIDO:
CROSS WRIST GRAB

TECHNIQUE #2

2a) The opponent grabs your wrist,
b) Reverse the opponent's grab using a small clockwise circular movement (grabbing his wrist) while sidestepping with your opposite foot,
c) and execute a rear vertical punch to the opponent's mid-section (yell on the punch).

Note: It is very important to sidestep far enough away from the opponent so that they can not reach you with their free

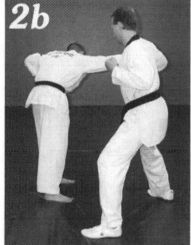

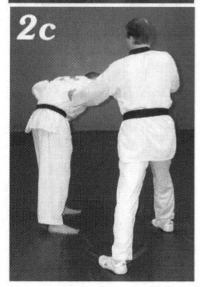

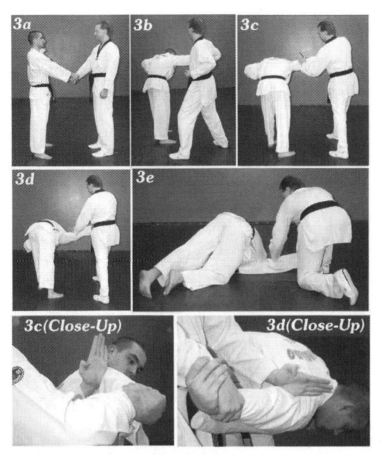

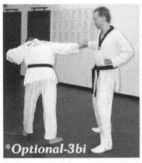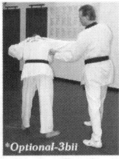

HAPKIDO:
CROSS WRIST GRAB

TECHNIQUE #3

3a) The opponent grabs your wrist,
b) Reverse the opponent's grab using a small clockwise circular movement (grabbing his wrist) while sidestepping with your opposite foot,
c-e) execute an arm-bar takedown using a knifehand (Yell on the takedown).

Note: Utilize the bone in your wrist to increase pain in the opponent's triceps muscle. This will encourage the opponent to go down to escape the pain.

Optional-3bi to 3bii
If your opponent tries to resist your arm-bar takedown execute an upper-cut to their rib-cage area to loosen them up. This is called a "Softening Up technique". Softening Up techniques are very important when dealing with large, strong, powerful opponent's. This will decrease their ability to resist your technique.

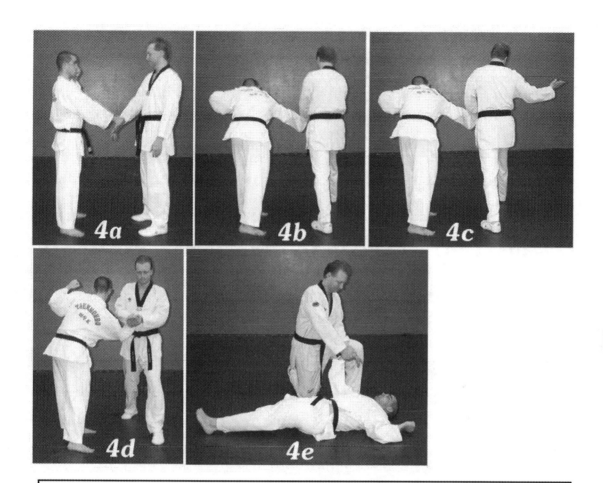

HAPKIDO:
CROSS WRIST GRAB

TECHNIQUE #4

4a) The opponent grabs your wrist,

b) With your free hand grab your opponent's hand to implement a wrist-lock while you simultaneously sidestep into a long walking stance,

c) Turn your palm up to twist out of your opponent's grip,

d) Use the hand that is now free to reinforce the wrist lock while simultaneously stepping out with your rear foot into another long walking stance in the opposite direction,

e) Twist your opponent's wrist making the palm of their hand face the floor while simultaneously executing a takedown by dropping to the knee that is closest to your opponent (yell on the take-down).

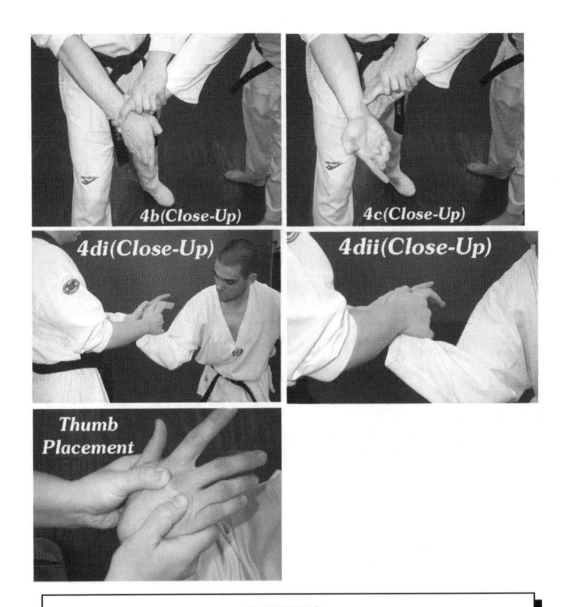

4b(Close-Up)

4c(Close-Up)

4di(Close-Up)

4dii(Close-Up)

Thumb Placement

HAPKIDO:
CROSS WRIST GRAB

TECHNIQUE #4(CLOSE-UP)

Note: In the above pictures 4b-4c study how the defender breaks out of the opponent's grip. Also take notice of how to position your thumbs on the opponent's hand as you are attempting to execute the wrist-lock.

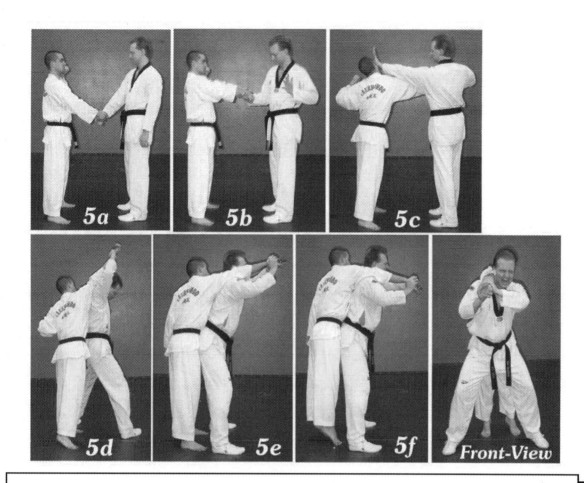

HAPKIDO:
CROSS WRIST GRAB

TECHNIQUE #5

5a) The opponent grabs your wrist,

b) Reverse the opponent's grip by grabbing on the inner side of opponent's wrist,

c) Pull them towards you while simultaneously executing a palm heel strike (using your free hand) to their temple,

d) Step under and through opponent's arm while simultaneously turning the opponent's palm up,

e) Reinforce your grip with your other hand and place the opponent's elbow slightly past your shoulder,

f) Pull the arm straight down breaking the opponent's elbow on your shoulder (yell on the elbow -break).

Note: Stretch out your opponent's arm for leverage by placing your buttocks right up against their hip while simultaneously pulling their arm out straight as in picture 5f.

Chapter Eleven

Single-Collar Grab Defenses

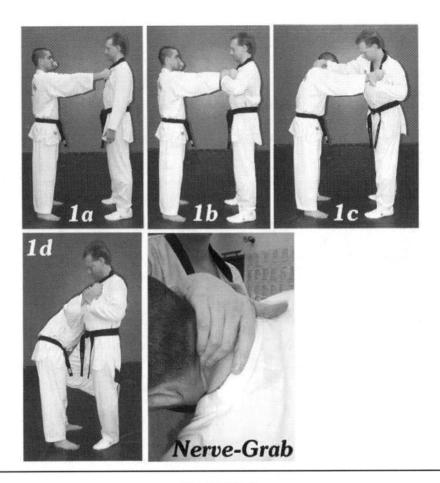

Nerve-Grab

TECHNIQUE #1

1a) The opponent grabs your collar,

b) Grab the opponent's wrist from the outside,

c) With your free hand hook the opponent behind their neck by digging your middle finger into the pressure/nerve point on the opposite side of their neck,

d) Pull the opponent in towards you and execute a knee strike to the groin (yell on the knee-strike).

Note: Some experimentation must done to find exactly where the opponent's nerve is located on the side of their neck. After much practice you should be able to find it immediately.

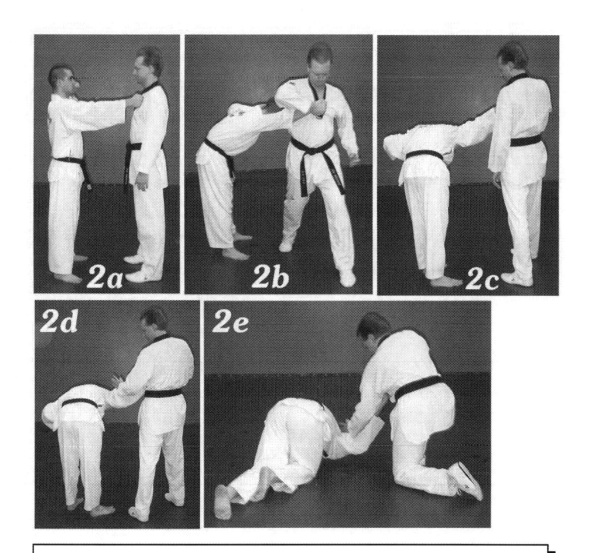

HAPKIDO:
SINGLE-COLLAR GRAB

TECHNIQUE #2

2a) The opponent grabs your collar,

b) Side step into a walking stance and reach across and grab the opponent's hand to set-up for a wrist-lock,

c) Twist back into a walking stance in the opposite direction while simultaneously applying the wrist lock,

d) Then lock out the opponent's elbow (utilizing a knifehand) and drop to the knee closest to your opponent taking them to the ground (yell on the take-down).

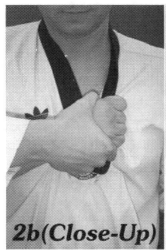

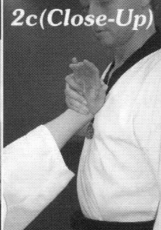

2c(Close-Up)

2b(Close-Up)

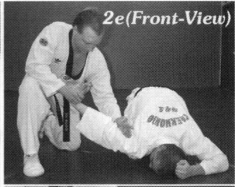

2e(Front-View)

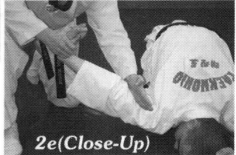

2e(Close-Up)

HAPKIDO:
SINGLE-COLLAR GRAB

TECHNIQUE #2(CLOSE-UP)

Note: Study the above pictures (2b-2c) to learn how to properly grab the opponent's hand to prepare for the wrist-lock. Utilize the bone in your wrist as you execute the knifehand to the opponent's triceps muscle to increase the pain.

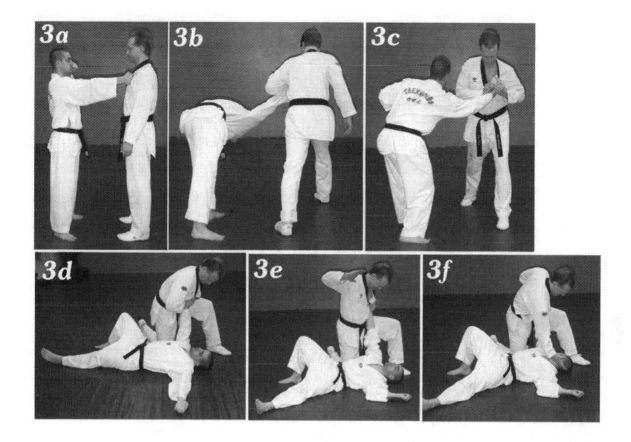

HAPKIDO:
SINGLE-COLLAR GRAB

TECHNIQUE #3

3a) The opponent grabs your collar,
b) Sidestep into a walking stance to get the opponent off balance while simultaneously grabbing the opponent's hand,
c) Use your opposite hand to reinforce for a double underhand wrist lock while sidestepping into another walking stance in the opposite direction,
d) To complete the takedown keep turning the wrist while making the opponent's hand face the ground while dropping to the knee that is closest to the opponent,
e-f) and execute a knifehand strike to the opponent's neck or head (yell on the knifehand strike).

Note: The outside hand does not let go while you are executing the knifehand strike to their throat.

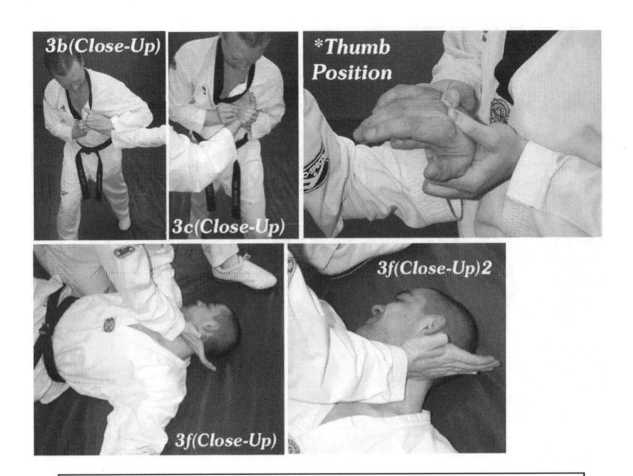

3b(Close-Up)

3c(Close-Up)

*Thumb Position

3f(Close-Up)2

3f(Close-Up)

HAPKIDO:
SINGLE-COLLAR GRAB

TECHNIQUE #3(CLOSE-UP)

Note: Study the finger and thumb positions used to set-up for the wrist-lock take down.

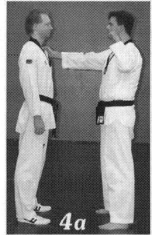

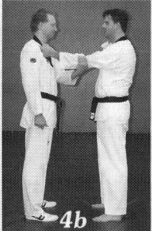

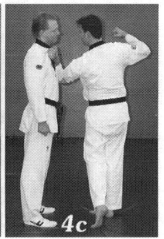

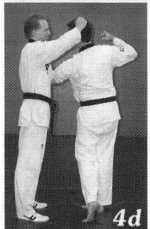

HAPKIDO:
SINGLE-COLLAR GRAB

TECHNIQUE #4

4a) The opponent grabs your collar,

b) Reach under the opponent's elbow (hooking nerve with two fingers),

c) Pull the opponent's elbow across in the opposite direction buckling the opponent's upper body inward,

d) With your free hand grab your opponent's hair at the crown,

e) Pivot 90-degrees and kneel down on the knee that is closest to the opponent,

f-g) Execute a knifehand strike to the opponent's head (yell on the strike).

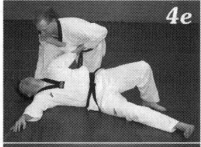

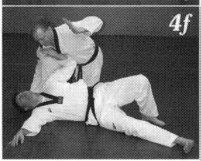

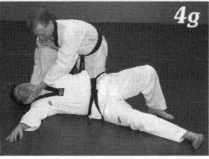

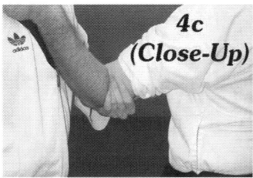

4c (Close-Up)

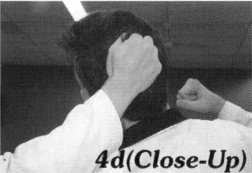

4d(Close-Up)

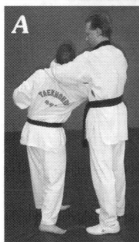

A

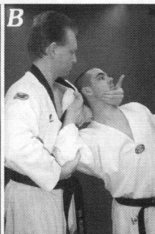

B

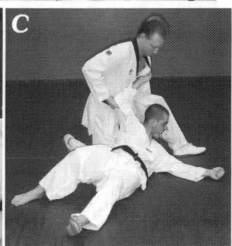

C

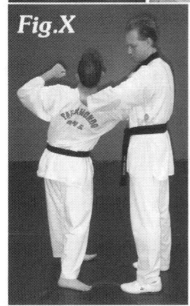

Fig.X

HAPKIDO:
SINGLE-COLLAR GRAB

TECHNIQUE #4
(OPTIONS)

Note: If your opponent does not have hair long enough to grab a hold of you can grab the opponent's jaw (Pics-A,B,C) or collar (Fig.X) for leverage. Also notice in Pic.4c(Close-Up) how to utilize the fingers in a hooking manner to control the opponent's elbow.

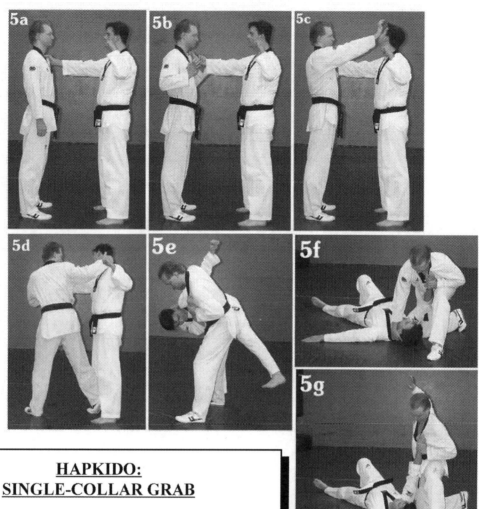

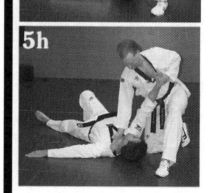

HAPKIDO:
SINGLE-COLLAR GRAB

TECHNIQUE #5

5a) The opponent grabs your collar,
b) Grab your opponent's wrist from the outside,
c) Execute a palm heel strike to the opponent's nose,
d) Step in between the opponent's feet as your free hand hooks behind opponents neck with a nerve grab,
e-f) Pivot 90-degrees on your foot that is in between your opponent's feet taking them to the ground by dropping to the knee that is closest to them,
g-h) and execute a knifehand strike to the opponent's neck of head (yell on the knifehand strike).

Note: Do not let go of the opponent's wrist while you execute the knifehand strike. If you do they might roll away and escape.

Chapter Twelve

Double-Collar Grab Defenses

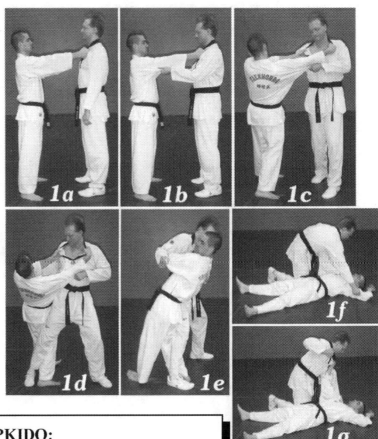

HAPKIDO:
DOUBLE-COLLAR GRAB

TECHNIQUE #1

1a) Your opponent grabs your collar,

b) Grab your opponent's sleeves at their elbows,

c) Steer your opponent by pulling with one hand pushing away with the other,

d) Step across and behind opponent's leg,

e) Push the opponent over your leg,

f) Take the opponent to the ground dropping to your knee that is closest to your opponent,

g-h) and execute a vertical punch to the opponent's head (yell on the vertical punch).

Note: One hand must be holding onto your opponent's sleeve as you execute the vertical punch to insure that they do not roll away or escape.

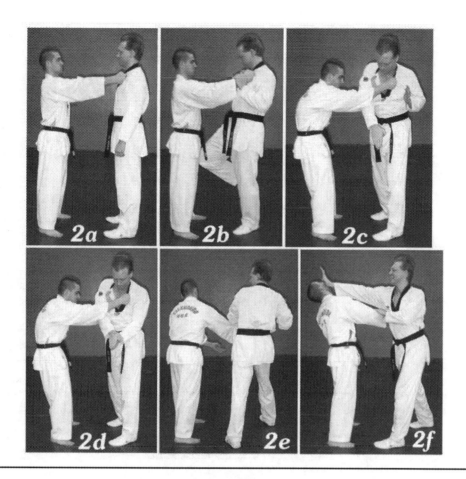

HAPKIDO:
DOUBLE-COLLAR GRAB

TECHNIQUE #2

2a) The opponent grabs your collar,

b) Grab both wrists of the opponent and execute an upward knee strike to the their groin,

c) Place one of your hands over and thru your opponent's arms,

d) Make a prayer (by placing both your hands together),

e) Twist in the opposite direction into a walking stance (breaking out of the opponent's hold),

f) and execute a reverse palm heel strike to nose (yell on the strike).

Note: Utilization of the hips is the key to power for breaking out of your opponent's grip, not the strength of your arms.

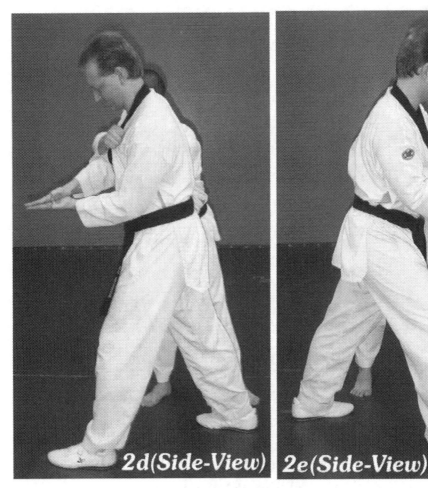
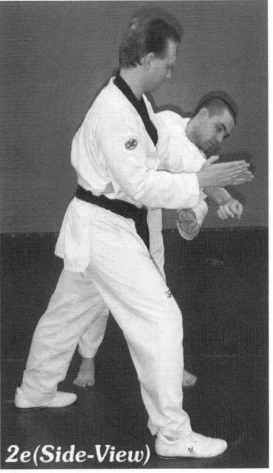

2d(Side-View) 2e(Side-View)

HAPKIDO:
DOUBLE-COLLAR GRAB

TECHNIQUE #2

Note: In the above pictures 2d and 2e notice how the hips are used for the defender's escape. The defender twists into a walking stance in one direction and then pivots 180-degrees into another walking stance.

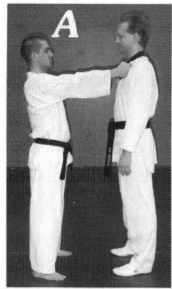

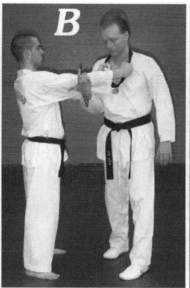

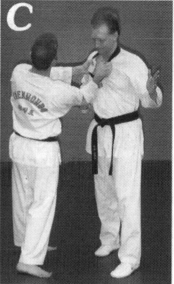

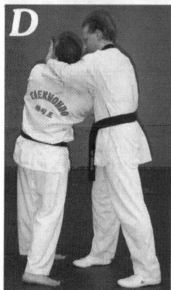

HAPKIDO:
DOUBLE-COLLAR GRAB

TECHNIQUE #3

A) The opponent grabs your collar,
B) Reach under and across to the opponent's opposite elbow,
C) Hook your fingers at the nerve pulling the opponent's elbow across to the side,
D) Grab the opponent's hair/jaw/or hair (at the crown),
E) With your knee that is closest to your opponent kneel down steering them to the ground,
F) and execute a knifehand strike to the opponent's neck (yell on the strike).

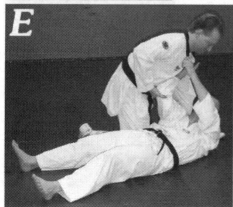

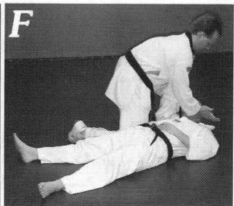

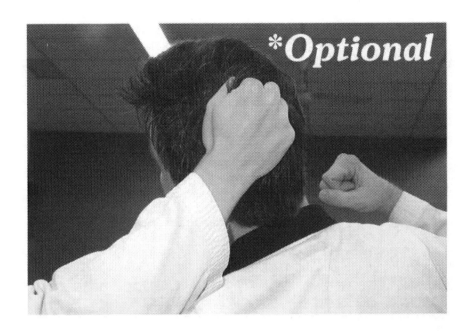

*Optional

HAPKIDO:
DOUBLE-COLLAR GRAB

TECHNIQUE #3(OPTIONAL)

Note: For this technique if the opponent has hair long enough to grab the best place is to utilize the hair at crown of the skull.

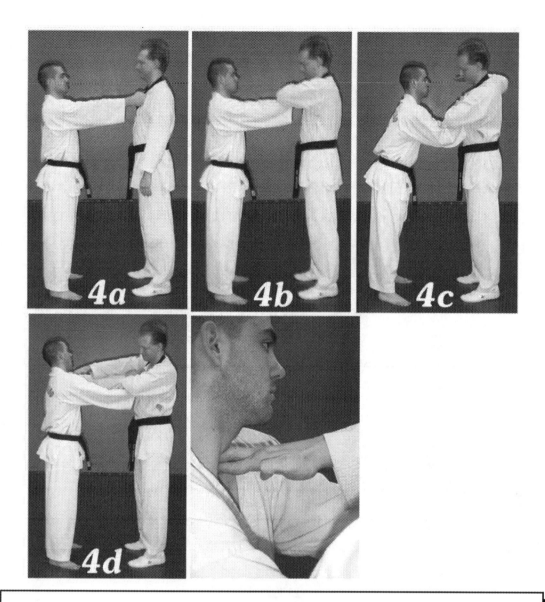

HAPKIDO:
DOUBLE-COLLAR GRAB

TECHNIQUE #4

4a) The opponent grabs your collar,

b) Reach over the top and grab the opponent's opposite wrist for control,

c-d) Execute a spear hand with your free hand to the opponent's throat while simultaneously stepping forward in between your opponent's legs (yell on the spear hand strike).

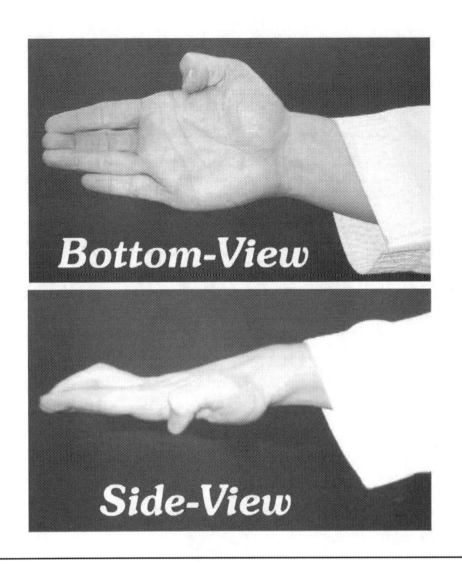

Bottom-View

Side-View

HAPKIDO:
DOUBLE-COLLAR GRAB

TECHNIQUE #4(CLOSE-UP)

Note: Strike with the three finger-tips between the thumb and pinky finger to execute a spear hand.

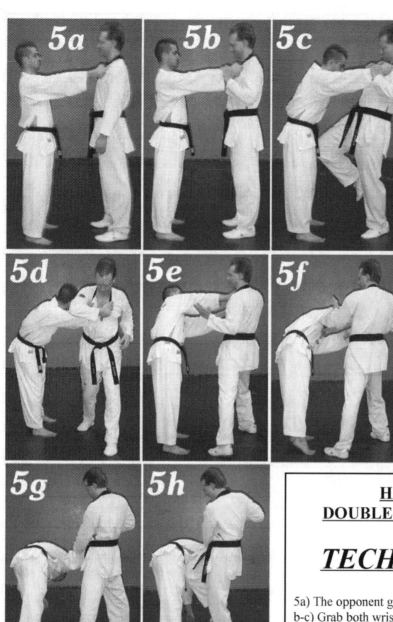

HAPKIDO:
DOUBLE-COLLAR GRAB

TECHNIQUE #5

5a) The opponent grabs your collar,
b-c) Grab both wrists of the opponent and execute an upward knee strike to the groin,
d) Reach across with the opposite hand while sidestepping into a walking stance while simultaneously grabbing the opponent's hand to implement an overhand wrist lock,
e-g) Implement an arm-bar by locking out the opponent's elbow with a knifehand behind the opponent's triceps muscle,
h) and execute an upward knee strike to opponents mid-section (yell on the knee strike).

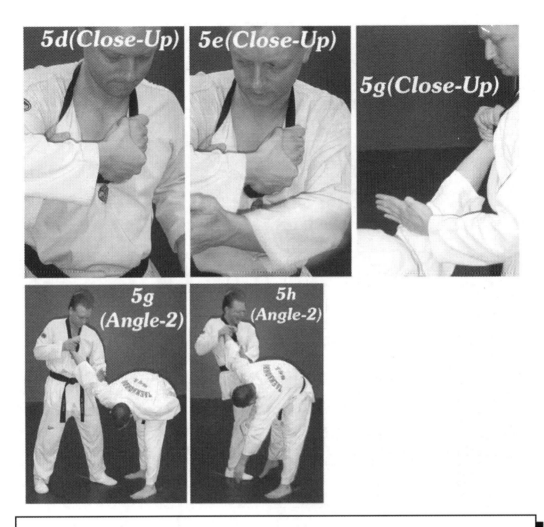

HAPKIDO:
DOUBLE-COLLAR GRAB

TECHNIQUE #5(CLOSE-UP)

Note: In order to implement the initiation of the wrist lock place your thumb between the opponent's thumb and index finger. Bending the wrist backwards as if you were trying to get the opponent's fingers to touch their elbow. Although they'll never reach(hopefully), that's your guide for perfect execution of this technique.

Chapter Thirteen

Side-Shoulder Grab Defenses

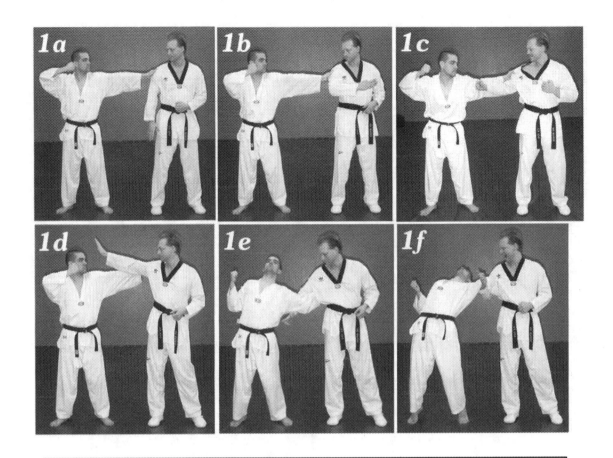

HAPKIDO:
SIDE-SHOULDER GRAB

TECHNIQUE #1

1a) The opponent grabs your shoulder,
b-c) Execute a backfist to the opponent's biceps muscle to loosen up the opponent's arm,
d-f) and execute a Snake-Lock to the opponent's elbow by guiding your forearm in a circular fashion behind their triceps muscle and point your fingers up towards the ceiling (yell on the Snake-Lock).

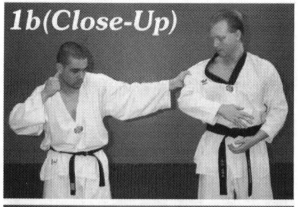

1b(Close-Up)

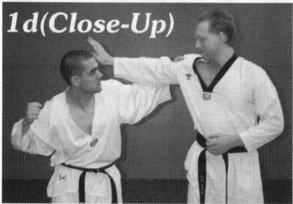

1d(Close-Up)

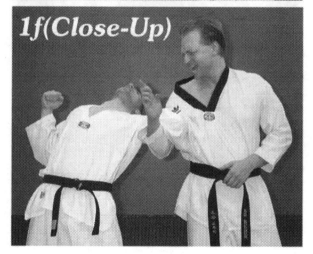

1f(Close-Up)

HAPKIDO:
SIDE-SHOULDER GRAB

TECHNIQUE #1 (CLOSE-UP)

Note: It is very important to make sure that your forearm goes past your opponent's elbow and touches their biceps muscle to properly implement the lock. Notice that as you point your finger upwards as in picture 1f (Close-up), the opponent's bent elbow turns upwards as well. Also observe that their spine arches. When you can see all these small details in your execution you will know that your technique is correct.

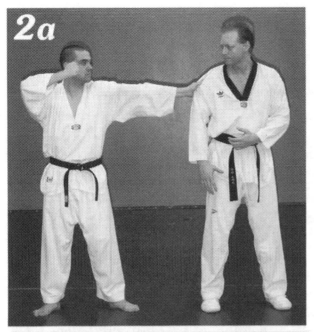

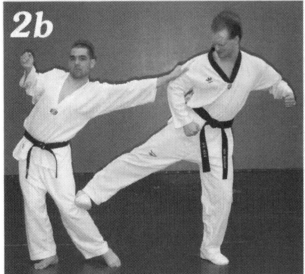

TECHNIQUE #2

2a) The opponent grabs your shoulder,
b) and execute a lead leg sidekick to the opponent's knee(yell on the sidekick).

Note: It is very important to drive your body weight into your opponent's knee. Put your hip into it. When practicing with a partner never actually make any contact to their knee. For practicing power use a low target like a low hanging punching bag.

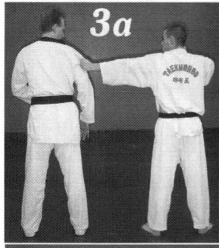

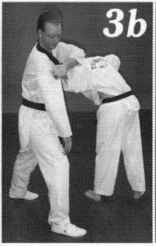

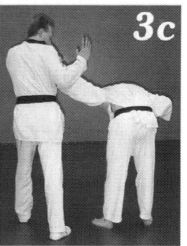

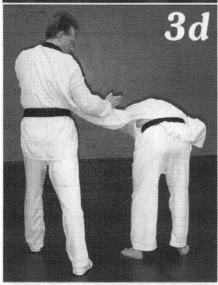

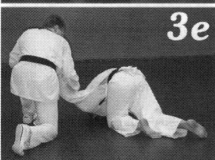

HAPKIDO:
SIDE-SHOULDER GRAB

TECHNIQUE #3

3a) The opponent grabs your shoulder,
b) With your opposite hand grab your opponent's hand (for an overhand wrist-lock) as you side-step towards your opponent's blindside (their back),
c-d) Pivot back 90-degrees and utilize a knifehand behind the opponent's elbow locking it out to implement an arm-bar,
e) Kneel down with your knee that is closest to your opponent and simultaneously take the opponent to the ground (yell on the takedown).

Note: Once again it is very important to use the bone in the wrist when using the knifehand to increase the amount of pain in the opponent's arm. This pain will greatly entice them to drop to the floor to escape the pain. Therefore "Action causes Reaction".

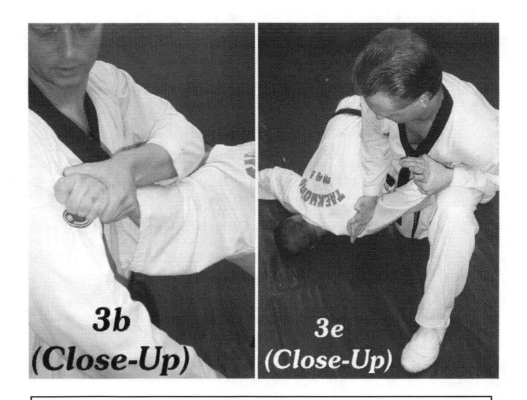

3b (Close-Up)

3e (Close-Up)

<u>HAPKIDO:
SIDE-SHOULDER GRAB</u>

TECHNIQUE #3(CLOSE-UP)

Note: Study the hand positions in the above pictures so that you can better understand the necessary mechanics for this technique.

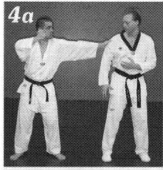 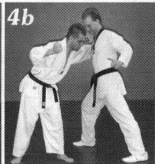 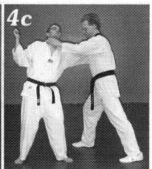

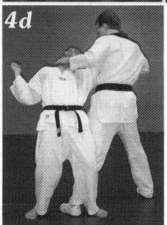

HAPKIDO:
SIDE-SHOULDER GRAB

TECHNIQUE #4

4a) The opponent grabs your shoulder,
b) Grab your opponent's wrist while simultaneously sidestepping into a walking stance facing your opponent,
c-d) With your rear foot step across and behind the lead leg of your opponent while your free hand grabs the throat of your opponent,
e) Push the opponent over your leg taking them to the ground,
f-g) Kneel down with the knee that is closest to your opponent and execute a vertical punch to the their head (yell on the vertical punch).

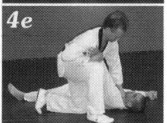

Note: Do not let go of the opponent's wrist as you are executing the vertical punch. If you let go they have a chance of rolling away, escaping or even worse, punching you back.

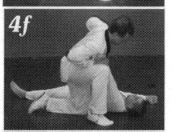

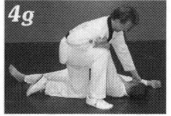

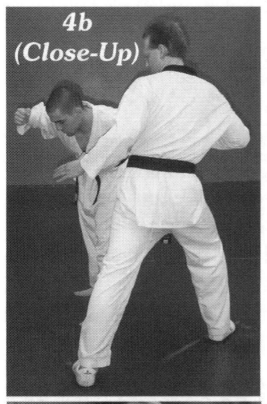

4b
(Close-Up)

HAPKIDO:
SIDE-SHOULDER GRAB

TECHNIQUE #4
(CLOSE-UP)

Note: When you grab your opponent's throat you can also strike them simultaneously. This hand position/technique is called a "tiger-mouth" strike. The striking area on your hand is between your index finger and your thumb. Tiger-mouth strikes are generally only used to the opponent's throat.

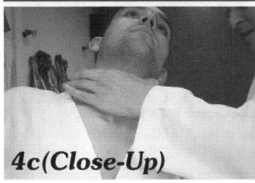

4c(Close-Up)

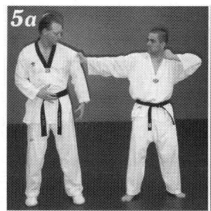
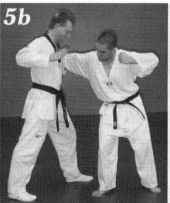
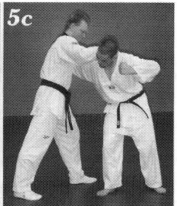

HAPKIDO:
SIDE-SHOULDER GRAB

TECHNIQUE #5

5a) The opponent grabs you shoulder,
b) Grab your opponent's wrist and sidestep into a walking stance,
c) With your opposite hand reach behind your opponent's neck (hooking the nerve with your two middle fingers),
d) Pull your opponent in towards you and execute an upward knee strike to their mid-section (yell on the knee strike).

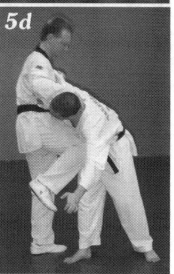

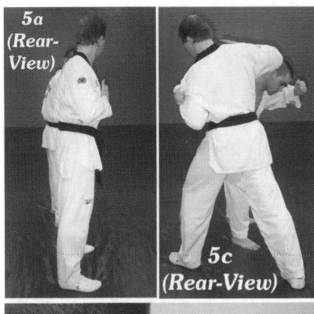

5a (Rear-View)

5c (Rear-View)

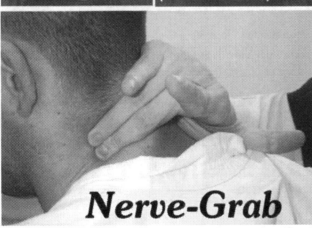

Nerve-Grab

HAPKIDO: SIDE-SHOULDER GRAB

TECHNIQUE #5 (REAR-VIEW)

Note: As you can see the great difference in body position relative to the opponent in pictures 5a-5c. It is very important to sidestep far enough to the opponent's blind-side to evade a possible attack from the opponent's free arm. Also notice the correct finger placement for the Nerve- Grab on the side of the opponent's neck. The two center fingers are used in a hooking fashion to dig in hard to inflict pain. This can cause an opponent to helplessly buckle inward making them more vulnerable during your counter attack.

Chapter Fourteen

Two-Handed Choke Defenses

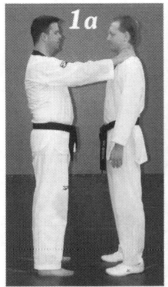 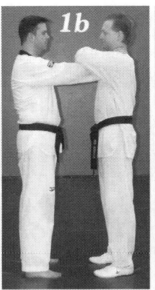 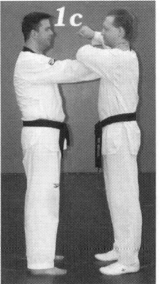

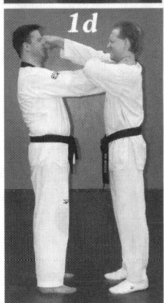

HAPKIDO:
TWO-HANDED CHOKE

TECHNIQUE #1

1a) The opponent grabs your throat,
b) Reach across and grab the opponent's opposite wrist,
c-d) and with your free hand execute an eye-gouge using your thumb.

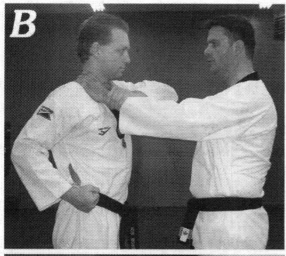

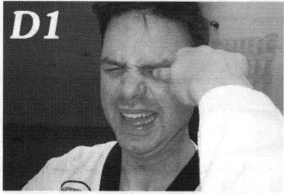

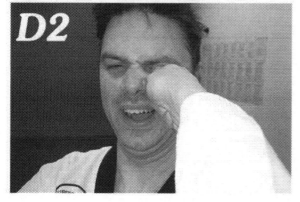

HAPKIDO:
TWO-HANDED CHOKE

TECHNIQUE #1 (CLOSE-UP)

Note: As you can see in picture B the opponent's wrist is trapped against the defender's body. The proper way to implement an eye gouge is demonstrated in pictures D1 and D2. The thumb is placed directly over the eye with the thumb nail facing the wall(or horizontal). The thumb is then turned upward in a corkscrew fashion making the thumbnail face the ceiling as it is gouged into the opponent's eye socket. Be careful not to make real contact with the eye when practicing in the dojo/dojang.

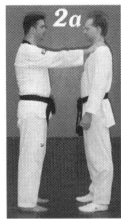
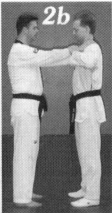
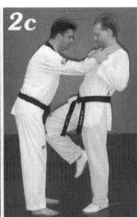
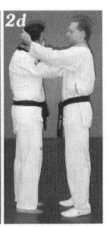

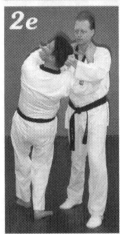

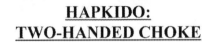

HAPKIDO:
TWO-HANDED CHOKE

TECHNIQUE #2

2a) The opponent grabs your throat,
b) Grab both wrists of the opponent,
c) Execute an upward knee-strike to groin,
d) With one hand grab the hair(at the crown) on back of the opponent's head while your other hand is placed on the side of the opponent's jaw using the heel of your palm,
e) Twist your opponent's head in the direction your palm is facing,
f) Take the opponent to the ground while simultaneously dropping to your knee that is closest to your opponent,
g-h) and execute a vertical punch to the opponent's head while holding the jaw wedged to the ground (yell on the vertical punch).

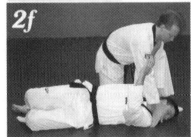

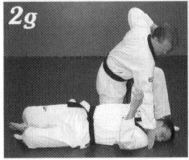

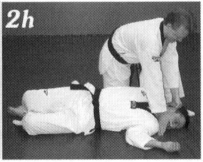

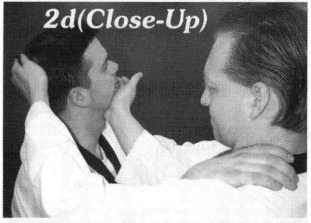

2d(Close-Up)

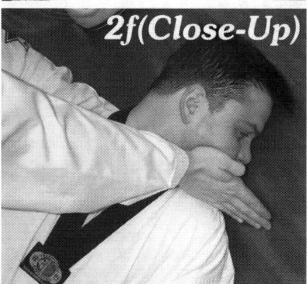

2f(Close-Up)

TECHNIQUE #2 (CLOSE-UP)

Note: For maximum control during the takedown study the hand positions used in the close-up picture 2d. In order to keep your opponent from getting up off the floor to retaliate against you, you must lean your whole body weight on their jaw as in close-up picture 2f.

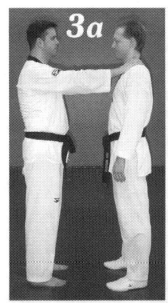
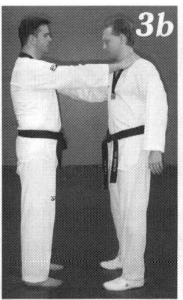
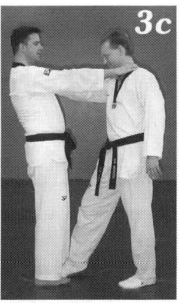

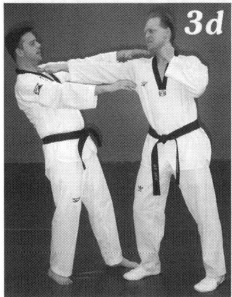

TECHNIQUE #3

3a) The opponent grabs your throat,
b-d) With your hand take the two fingers closest to your thumb and push on the opponent's wind pipe by coming up between the opponent's arms while simultaneously stepping forward between your opponent's legs.

Note: To increase the effectiveness of the technique drive your fingers deep into the wind pipe of the opponent(yell on the finger thrust).

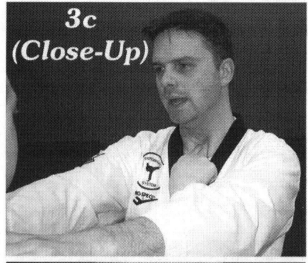

3c
(Close-Up)

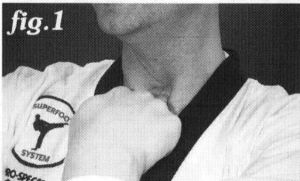

fig.1

TECHNIQUE #3 (CLOSE-UP)

Note: As demonstrated in pictures 3c(Close-Up) and fig.1 the proper placement of the fingers are on the hole in the neck just below the "Adam's Apple".

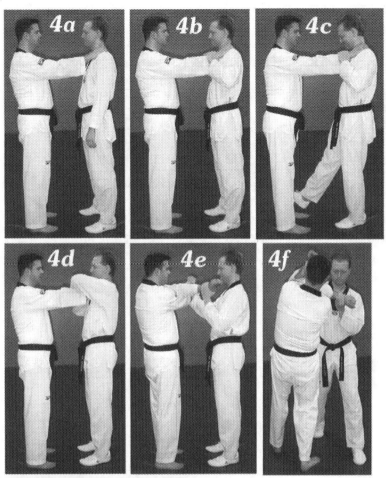

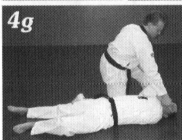

HAPKIDO:
TWO-HANDED CHOKE

TECHNIQUE #4

4a) The opponent grabs your throat,

b) Grab both wrists of the opponent,

c) Execute a front kick to the opponent's shin (using the ball of the foot),

d) With one hand reach over top and grab the opponent's opposite wrist while your opposite hand grabs underneath for the opponent's opposite wrist,

e-f) Pivot 180-degrees and twist the opponent's arms using the opponent's bottom arm to lock out opponent's top arm(elbow),

g) Drop to the knee that is closest to your opponent as you take them to the ground (yell on the take-down).

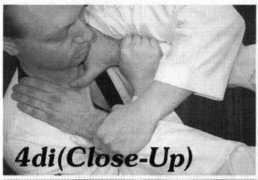

4di(Close-Up)

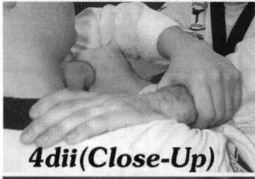

4dii(Close-Up)

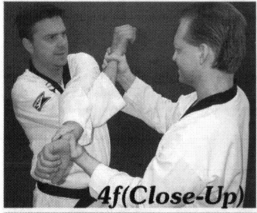

4f(Close-Up)

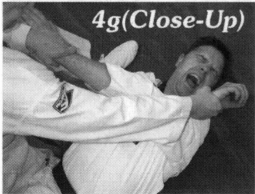

4g(Close-Up)

TECHNIQUE #4
(CLOSE-UP)

Note: Because of the complexity of this technique it is important to study the hand grips/positions to initiate the counter attack as seen in pictures 4di) and 4dii). Also take notice of the close-up pictures 4f) and 4g) so that you can learn to how to manipulate the opponent's arms to implement the elbow-lock takedown. Remember the opponent's forearm must be placed behind their opposite elbow in order to achieve a full functionality of this technique.

123

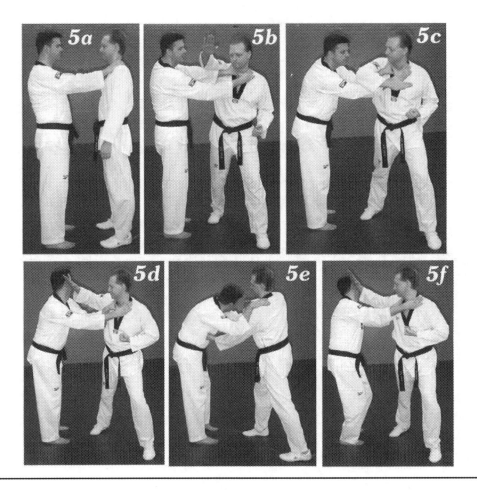

HAPKIDO:
TWO-HANDED CHOKE

TECHNIQUE #5

5a) Grab your opponent's throat,

b-c) With one arm trap your opponent's arms against your own chest and simultaneously position yourself in a walking stance facing 90-degrees to your opponent,

d) Execute a knifehand chop to the opponent's head/face/neck,

e) Retract your knifehand chop to chamber position while simultaneously executing an undercut punch to the opponent's rib-cage,

f) and execute another knifehand chop to opponent's head/face/neck area(yell on the last knifehand chop).

Note: When the proper mechanics of this technique are fully developed, then the student's next goal is to achieve blinding speed when releasing the combination hand strike.

Chapter Fifteen

Headlock
Defenses

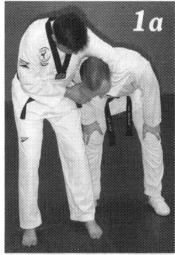 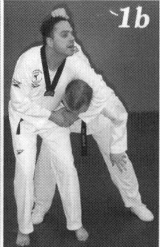 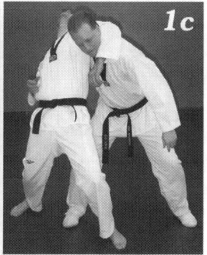

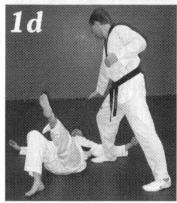

HAPKIDO:
HEADLOCK DEFENSES

TECHNIQUE #1

1a) The opponent attacks with a side headlock,
b) With the foot that is closest to the opponent step behind their closest leg wedging it behind their knee while with your hand that is closest to your opponent reach and grab the front of the opponent's hair (above the forehead),
c-d) Step back and simultaneously pull their hair straight back taking the opponent to the ground (yell on the take-down).

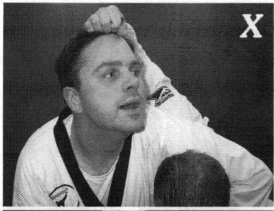

X

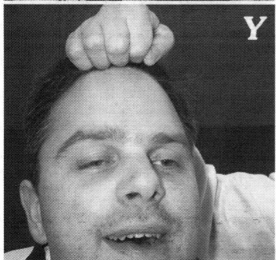

Y

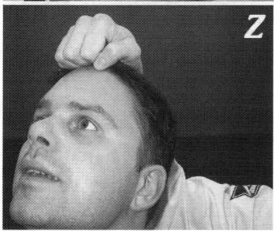

Z

HAPKIDO:
HEADLOCK DEFENSES

TECHNIQUE #1
CLOSE-UP

Note: It is very important to know how to exactly grab the opponent's hair to maintain maximum power and control during the technique. If the opponent is bald or has really short hair that you can not grab a hold of, just place the knife-edge of a knifehand across the bridge of the opponent's nose and push hard against the cartiledge. This will force the opponent to either fall down or at least release you from their grip. The pressure felt inside the nose will entice the opponent to release their grip because it feels like the nose is going to break or be crushed. Generally the opponent will try to move in the direction in which you are pushing the knifehand to escape the pain. This is your opportunity to direct them to the ground.

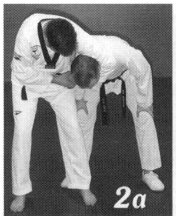
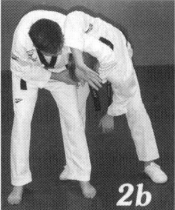
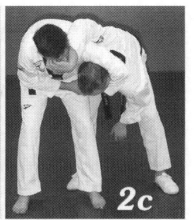
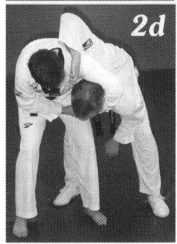

HAPKIDO:
HEADLOCK DEFENSES

TECHNIQUE #2

2a) The opponent attacks with a side headlock,
b) With the hand that is closest to the opponent reach across the opponent's face,
c-d) and execute a tiger-claw tearing across the opponent's face (yell on the tiger-claw).

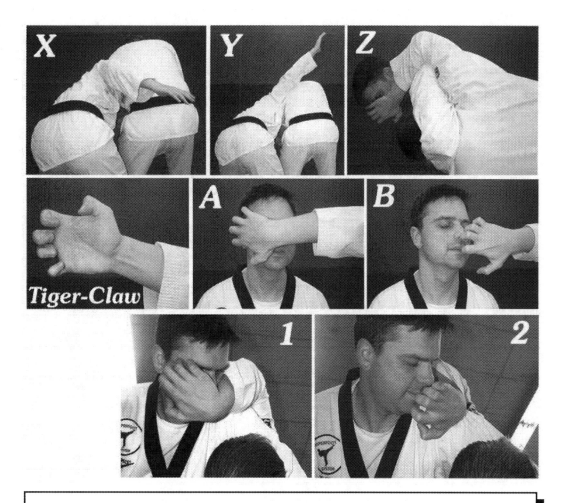

HAPKIDO:
HEADLOCK DEFENSES

TECHNIQUE #2

Note: Study the above close-up pictures to gain a better understanding of how to gain access to the opponent's face while in the side headlock position. Also notice the finger position that is used for the "Tiger-Claw". You are literally raking your finger nails across your opponent's face tearing at their skin to entice them to let go of their grip. If you can tear across their eyes in the process, you will find that this will really enhance your ability to escape the opponent's head-lock.

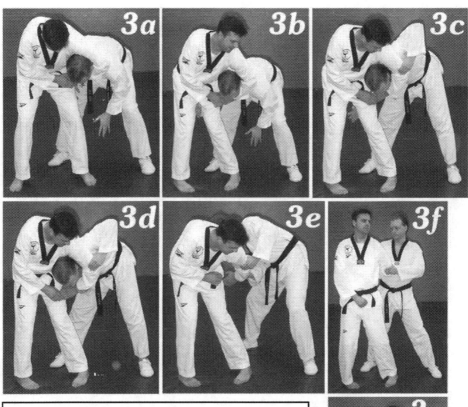

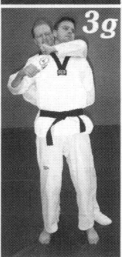

HAPKIDO:
HEADLOCK DEFENSES

TECHNIQUE #3

3a) The opponent attacks with a side headlock,
b) With the hand that is closest to your opponent execute a ridgehand to the opponent's groin from behind,
c) With your outside hand grab the nerve in the opponents elbow (pinch hard utilizing the thumb),
d-f) Pull the elbow outward and pull your head out as you grab the opponent's wrist with the hand closest to your opponent and with your outside hand apply a wrist-lock,
f) Gain control from behind (restraining the opponent) putting them into a combo wrist and head lock (yell on the restraining hold).

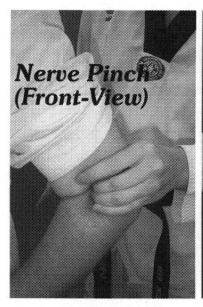

Nerve Pinch (Front-View)

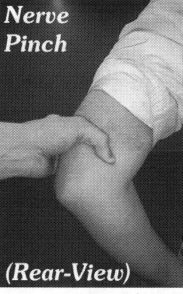

Nerve Pinch

(Rear-View)

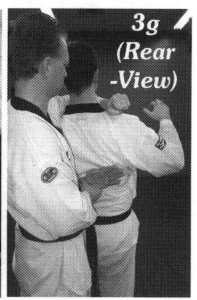

3g (Rear-View)

TECHNIQUE #3
(CLOSE-UP)

Note: In the above pictures which demonstrate the nerve pinch study how the fingers and thumb are used to control the opponent's elbow. Also take notice in picture 3g(Rear-View) that the defender leans back slightly to keep the attacker off balance. Leaning back for enough so that the opponent's weight is on their heels will allow you to properly restrain your opponent.

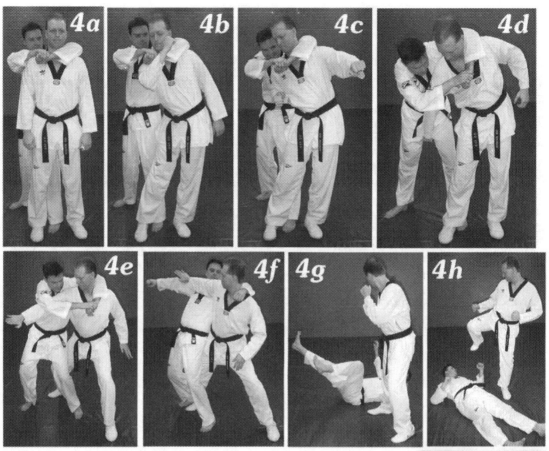

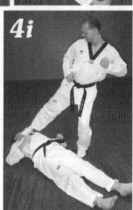

HAPKIDO:
HEADLOCK DEFENSES

TECHNIQUE #4

4a) The opponent attacks with a rear-headlock,

b) Twitch your buttocks away from the opponent exposing their mid-section and the groin,

c) Execute a rear elbow strike to the opponent's mid-section,

d) Execute a hammer fist to the opponent's groin,

e) With the foot that is closest to the opponent step in behind their closest leg going into a solid horse stance while simultaneously placing your arm across their chest,

f) With the same arm reach across the opponent's chest pushing them over your leg throwing them to the ground,

g) Execute a lead leg sidekick to the opponent's body or head after they have fallen to the ground (yell on the sidekick).

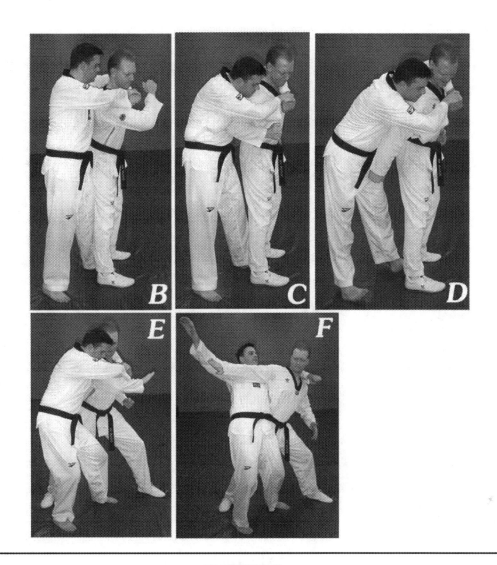

TECHNIQUE #4
(SIDE-VIEW)

Note: It is very important to keep your knees bent while throwing your opponent over your leg. If your leg is too straight you can cause serious damage to your knee joint depending on the weight of your opponent. The heavier the opponent, the more danger your knees are in if you do not keep them properly bent.

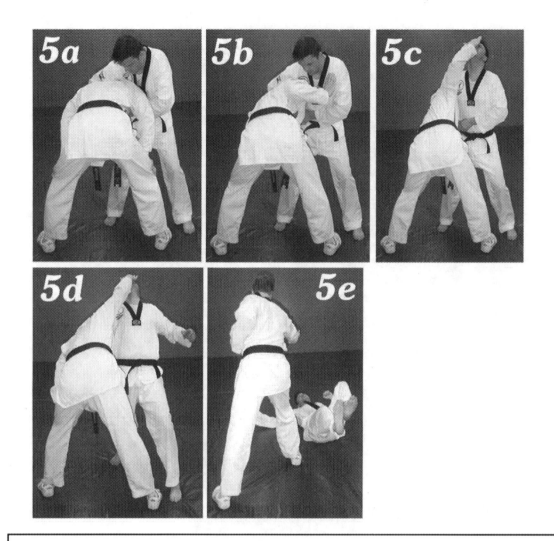

HAPKIDO:
HEADLOCK DEFENSES

TECHNIQUE #5

5a) The opponent attacks with reverse side headlock,
b-e) With the hand that is closest to your opponent execute a palm heel strike to the opponent's nose(yell on the palm heel strike).

Note: For safe practice in the dojo/dojang place the heel of your palm on the bridge of the opponent's nose and push gently forcing the opponent backward due to the pressure caused in the nose. The opponent will feel forced into releasing their grip due to the fact that it will feel as if their nose is going to break or be crushed.

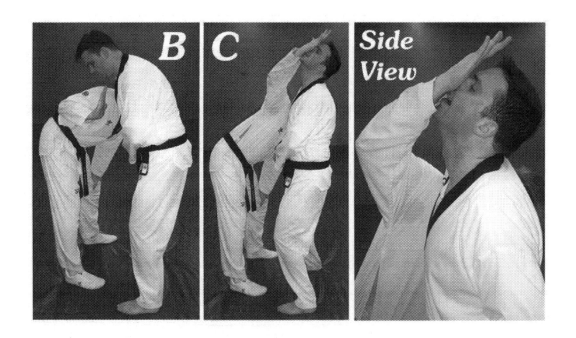

HAPKIDO:
HEADLOCK DEFENSES

TECHNIQUE #5
(SIDE-VIEW)

Note: For extra power in your movement it is important to step forward in between your opponent's feet as you execute the palm heel strike to their nose.

Chapter Sixteen

Martial Arts Videos and Books

by Adam Gibson

Martial Art Videos and Books
by Adam Gibson

Item #068

Scientific Speed Training (Best-Seller)

A revolutionary new video that is guaranteed to improve your speed in combat. Speed in combat is much more complex than how fast you can punch or kick from point-A to point-B. In fact there are different types of speed which are: 1) PHYSICAL SPEED) 2) SPEED OF TECHNIQUE 3) SPEED OF REACTION TIME. Also there are methods that can slow down your opponent's thinking (reaction-time) in essence making you faster. Scientifically enhance your speed through proven exercises and drills professional fighters are using around the world. Another advantage of these training methods are the ability to beat an opponent to the punch or kick even if they are physically faster than you. Speed is one of the most important aspects of fighting so don't be without this vital knowledge.

$39.95 U.S./$ 63.00 Canadian

Item #042

1000 Counter-Attacks (Best-Seller)

1000 Counter-Attacks is the only video tape on earth to bring you ONE THOUSAND DIFFERENT TECHNIQUES that were designed to be used while on the defensive. This video is like no other. We show defenses against every major kick, punch, and strike used in martial arts today. For example you'll learn how to counter: FRONT KICKS ROUNDHOUSE KICKS, SIDEKICKS ,TURN-BACK KICKS,SPIN-KICKS, JUMP-KICKS, AXE-KICKS, JABS REVERSE PUNCHES, HOOK PUNCHES, RIDGEHAND STRIKES, BACKFIST ATTACKS and COMBINATION ATTACKS. Also we show how to defend yourself when your opponent attacks with LEAD-LEG or REAR-LEG kicks and whether you and your opponent are in an OPEN-STANCE or a CLOSED-STANCE. In the last portion of the video we have an excellent KNIFE and GUN SECTION perfect for anyone who wishes to improve their chances in a street confrontation. All in all the information on this tape surpasses any video on the market today! A TOTAL STEAL!
APPROXIMATE RUNNING TIME: 4 HOURS 18 MINUTES.

$39.95 U.S./$ 63.00 Canadian

Item
#048

Offensive Footwork (Volume 1)

This videotape demonstrates the most commonly used offensive footwork drills used by top competitors today. Watch Mr. Gibson step-for-step as he breaks down each piece of footwork and explains its purpose. The best way to attack your opponent is knowing what footwork to use in any given situation.

$29.95 U.S/$47.00 Canadian

Item
#049

Offensive Footwork (Volume 2)

This videotape demonstrates how to use offensive footwork in a sparring or tournament situation. The drills on this tape will develop your ability to instinctively select the proper footwork to attack your opponent with. Whether your opponent is in an open-stance or closed-stance, close range or far range with reference to you, this video will show you how to go about commencing your attack scientifically with minimal worries of being countered on entry. An excellent addition to any serious competitors library.

$29.95 U.S/$47.00 Canadian

Item
#050

Defensive Footwork (Volume 1)

This videotape will enhance the martial artist's ability to develop the proper footwork skills while on the defensive. Depending on how deep the opponent attacks will decide which type of footwork will be used. The drills on this tape will teach the fighter footwork that can be applied from close to far range situations.

$29.95 U.S/$47.00 Canadian

Item
#051

Defensive Footwork (Volume 2)

This video will show the martial artist how to combine his or her defensive footwork with punch and kick counter-attacks, the ability to move and counter is an entire art in itself. Through the drills on this tape you will develop superior timing (decreased reaction time) and excellent technical skills for the ring.

$29.95 U.S/$47.00 Canadian

Item
#052

Angular Footwork (Offensive and Defensive)

This videotape will show the martial artist how to attack and defend utilizing precise angles to flank the opponent and to avoid getting hit. Everybody knows how to attack in a straight line!! Most martial arts only teach attacking in a straight line!! They also on the average teach defending in a straight line!! Remember, one of the keys of beating an opponent who's more experienced than you, is to use techniques or strategies that he or she has never seen. In this tape we offer that information.

$29.95 U.S/$47.00 Canadian

Item
#053

Set-Ups (Using Footwork)

Learn how to set-up your opponent using scientifically designed footwork drills that will open up your opponent's defenses. Footwork can be one of the most devastating tools in combat or sparring. In martial arts footwork has been unfortunately avoided, overlooked, and under-rated. This is because science is involved for effective footwork. If you don't understand something you throw it aside until someone shows you how to do it, or you figure it out yourself. Don't fear, someone has already figured it out for you and can show you the drills and science behind setting-up your opponent with the use of footwork. I urge you to purchase this one of a kind video that will change your entire perspective of fighting.

$29.95 U.S/$47.00 Canadian

Item
#054

Lateral Footwork (Applications)

This video concentrates on uses for lateral footwork for advanced sparring. When you can't get a bead on your opponent sparring in a straight line (which most people only know how to do) use lateral footwork to set-up an opening. Lateral footwork can be applied whether your on the offense or the defense. The drills on this tape will show you how to attack and defend with ease using lateral footwork methods. Lateral footwork can also be used against weapons, which we also have a section on this tape for. It's up to you to get the edge that most fighters don't have. That edge is knowledge.

$29.95 U.S/$47.00 Canadian

Item
#056

Super Footwork Drills (Single or Partner Training)

The best type of drills in martial arts are drills which can be done with or without a partner. Solo-training can be one of the most productive training methods in a martial artist's arsenal, while partner training is an unavoidable part of martial arts in order to become the best. The exercises on this tape are designed for both. Learn how to be super-smooth in the ring. Attack without fear of being hit. Counter-attack with safety. This video is for the advanced martial artist or master level practitioner who wishes to master his or her skills in the art of mobility.

$29.95 U.S/$47.00 Canadian

Item
#057

The Art of Faking: Principles and Concepts (Volume-1)

Martial arts or combat is much more complex than just kick-punch or attack-defend. In order to land a punch or kick effectively against a trained fighter one must have solid strategies based on science. The art of faking is one of those solid strategies. There are four different ways of faking: 1) Footwork, 2) Combinations, 3) Head & body movement, and 4) Mental programming. Don't be without this extremely important strategy. It could change your whole outlook on fighting.

Item #058

The Art of Faking: Kicking (Volume-2)

In our second volume one the art of faking we specialize on how to set-up your opponent using your kicks only. The three types of techniques demonstrated on this tape are: 1) Lead-leg set-ups 2) Probe kick set-ups and 3) Counter-attack luring. Each section shows scientifically designed strategies which force your opponent to react in different ways. Depending how your opponent reacts will decide what your next move will be. Just think, if you could position your opponent's head, body, feet, guards and mental focus exactly the way you wanted you probably would hit your opponent at will. Learn the techniques that only master fighters and top competitors use and you too can be the best.

$29.95 U.S/$47.00 Canadian

Item #059

The Art of Faking: Kicking and Punching (Volume-3)

Very few martial artists know how to effectively use their hands and feet as an entire unit. By practicing the techniques on this tape, you'll learn how to correctly and deceptively fake, with either your hands or feet to open up your opponent's defenses and score with ease. Any time you kick or punch you cause a reaction in your opponent, whether it is mentally and physically or just mentally. Learn to improve your sparring 3-fold by learning these advanced strategies.

$29.95 U.S/$47.00 Canadian

Item #064

Jamming: Short Circuit Your Opponent's Movements

What's one of the best ways to neutralize an opponent's weapons? Jamming. Jamming is used to smother or block deflect an opponents weapons. Also some forms of counter-attacking can be considered as a form of jamming. An example would be a stopping sidekick to an opponents back-leg roundhouse kick attack. You stick that sidekick between you and your opponent before they can complete their kick. So therefore you just neutralized the opponent's weapon. The techniques on this video can be applied in far, medium and close-range situations. We also show jamming as a weapon of attack and defense. Just think, if an opponent can't get his kick or his punch out, how can he beat you? Learn to attack without fear and to defend with confidence!

$29.95 U.S/$47.00 Canadian

Item #070

Endurance: How to Obtain Maximum Endurance

In combat your endurance can be your best friend or worst enemy. A more experienced fighter or even a champion can be beaten by an opponent with a higher endurance level and with much less experience. The advantages of high levels of endurance are: {1) Improved Circulation To The Muscles, 2) Improved Muscle Coordination, 3) Enhanced Speed, 4) Elimination Of Sluggishness, 5) Improved Energy, 6) Higher Pain Threshold, 7) Improved Focus (Alertness), 8) Improved Ability To Overcome Unforeseen Obstacles Quicker and More.. Obviously the above advantages are not just advantages for combat, but for ordinary everyday life. Martial arts benefits are designed not just to develop one physically, but they are to enhance oneself mentally, spiritually, and emotionally. High endurance training is one of the best ways, if not the only way, to reach the highest levels of martial arts prowess and discipline. Practice the training regiments on this tape and develop yourself into the martial artist you've always dreamed of being.

$29.95 U.S/$47.00 Canadian

Item #071

The Deadly Sidekick: Master the Most Powerful Kick in Combat

In the martial arts the most powerful kick is the sidekick. It is a kick that can be used as an offensive and defensive weapon. What most martial artists don't realize is that you don' t need a hundred deadly kicks to be the best. You need only one. The catch is that you need to learn how to use that one kick a hundred different ways so that you can deal with any situation at any time. On this videotape we show all variations of the side kick and training methods. Footwork drills, attacking drills and counter-attacking drills are all included on this tape. The sidekick is a preferred weapon by top martial artists; like Bruce Lee, Joe Lewis and Bill Wallace. The reason for this is that it is a very functional kick. This is the only tape ever designed that is solely dedicated to developing the sidekick. Enhance your skills with this unique training video.

$29.95 U.S/$47.00 Canadian

Item
#077

Joint-Locks: How to Control Your Opponent

In a self-defense situation, one of the best ways to control your opponent is through the use of joint-lock techniques. Joint-lock techniques can be used when an opponent tries to punch you, grab you, stab or club you and also while holding a gun to your head or body. On this tape you will learn to implement the following: 1) WRIST-LOCKS, 2) ELBOW-LOCKS, 3) SHOULDER-LOCKS, and 4) HEAD-LOCKING STYLE MANEUVERS Using these techniques, you will learn to defend yourself from the following: 1)WRIST-GRABS 2) COLLAR-GRABS 3) CHOKES 4) SHOULDER-GRABS 5) KNIFE-ATTACKS 6) GUN ATTACKS.
This Is One Of The Most Complete Joint-Lock Tapes Available On The Market Today!!!

$29.95 U.S/$47.00 Canadian

Item
#087

Super Leg Conditioning: Endurance, Strength, Flexibility, and Agility

Learn all you need to know about conditioning your legs for competition and all around combat. *Develop MUSCULAR ENDURANCE that will allow you to kick fifteen (15) rounds (or more) for full-contact events which demand such fitness. *Develop increased amounts of strength in your legs which allow you to kick with more POWER and LEG-CONTROL. *Develop the FLEXIBILITY needed to kick to the head with KNOCK-OUT POWER to an opponent who is taller than you are. *Develop EXTRAORDINARY AGILITY to out-maneuver any opponent to either attack or counter-attack. This video will become your bible on how to condition your legs for brutal combat. Don' t Be Without It!!

$29.95 U.S/$47.00 Canadian

Item
#088

Control Kicking: Kick 10 Times or More Without Dropping your Foot to the Ground

This video will show you the drills necessary to allow you to kick ten (10) times or more, head-level, without dropping your foot to the ground. Balance and coordination drills are highly emphasized on this tape to give you maximum control over your kicking leg. Advanced kicking combinations require this tape of skill, especially for fighter's who rely mostly on their lead-leg. Sometimes there isn' t time to drop your foot and then kick. This is where control kicking drills will give you the edge. Superior leg control also affects power and speed. The drills on this tape will provide you with an excellent work-out as well. An excellent choice for the martial artist who is continually upgrading his skills in the ring.

$29.95 U.S/$47.00 Canadian

Item
#091

How to Close the Gap: Covers Footwork and Distancing

In combat, one of the hardest things to do is to effectively close the gap. Closing the gap is to cover a given distance and be close enough to hit your opponent. Ever notice that when people spar, they miss way more than they score, when they attack. This is because there are more variables than meets the eye. This video will teach you drills on how to effectively close the gap for the most common situations in sparring. These situations could be as follows: If you and your opponent are in open or closed stances. If you are at close range, medium rang, or far range. If your opponent is an excellent counter-attacker. If your opponent always runs away as soon as you attack (or disengages). This is another excellent addition for the advanced competitor, who wishes to increase the quality of their sparring skills.

$29.95 U.S/$47.00 Canadian

Item
#092

The Art of Evasion: If They Can't Hit You, They Can't Beat You!!!

In my school I teach the students that defense is number one. Reason - because even if you're attacking you still have to protect yourself from being counter-attacked. So, what it comes down to, is that you always have to be defensive, whether you're the defender or the attacker. The art of evasion will teach you the skills to avoid any blow utilizing footwork and head/body movement. The drills on this tape are the most effective techniques of evasion to date and will have you slipping, ducking, and sidestepping your opponents in no time. Remember, the one who usually loses is the one who always gets hit. Take advantage of this wealth of information and baffle all opponents.

$29.95 U.S/$47.00 Canadian

Item
#093

Telegraphing: Learn to Predict Your Opponent's Moves!!!

Whenever an opponent throws a punch or kick, he leaves a clue of what technique he is throwing before he can finish. This is called telegraphing. This video will teach you how to recognize a telegraphic movement and take advantage. The whole concept of defense based on this tape will sharpen your awareness and increase your reaction time dramatically. Professional fighters use the same type of drills to perfect their defensive skills. From this video, you will learn how to defend yourself from punches and kicks effectively using science. Never fear to walk into the ring again, armed with the knowledge of how to read your opponent before they strike.

$29.95 U.S/$47.00 Canadian

Item
#110

NEW!!
SPORT KARATE -Volume #1
(Defensive Tactics)

In this video you will learn how to scientifically defend yourself from just about any type of attack used in Point Competition Sparring today. Learn where your opponent is open to score on when they attack with any punch or kick. Short-circuit your opponent's combination attacks with advanced footwork and jamming techniques. ***Dozens and dozens of defensive techniques on this tape are currently being used by top fighters and elite level competitors around the world.***

29.95 U.S.Funds/$47.00 Canadian

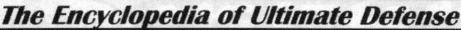
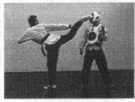 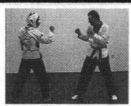 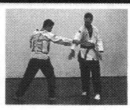 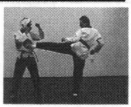
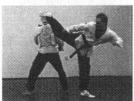 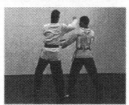 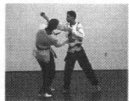 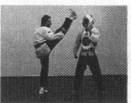
148

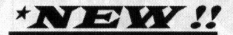
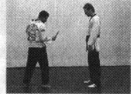
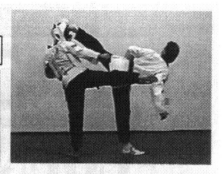
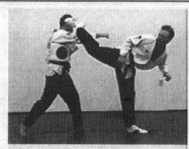
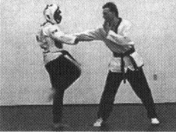
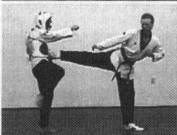
149

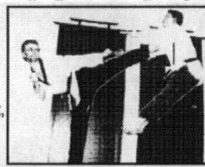

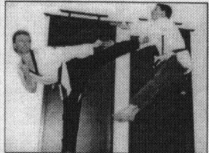

THE SCIENTIFIC VIDEO COLLECTION

BUY 3 or MORE VIDEOS and RECEIVE THE WHOLESALE-DISCOUNT of $19.95 U.S. per/Tape

TAPE#   **DESCRIPTION**

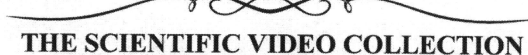

068 -SCIENTIFIC SPEED TRAINING (BEST-SELLER)
042 -1000 COUNTER-ATTACKS (BEST-SELLER)
048 -OFFENSIVE FOOTWORK (VOLUME 1)
049 -OFFENSIVE FOOTWORK (VOLUME 2)
050 -DEFENSIVE FOOTWORK (VOLUME 1)
051 -DEFENSIVE FOOTWORK (VOLUME 2)
052 -ANGULAR FOOTWORK (OFFENSIVE and DEFENSIVE)
053 -SET-UPS (USING FOOTWORK)
054 -LATERAL FOOTWORK (APPLICATIONS)
056 -SUPER FOOTWORK DRILLS (SINGLE or PARTNER TRAINING)
057 -THE ART OF FAKING: PRINCIPLES and CONCEPTS (VOLUME 1)
058 -THE ART OF FAKING: KICKING (VOLUME 2)
059 -THE ART OF FAKING: KICKING and PUNCHING (VOLUME 3)
064 -JAMMING: SHORT CIRCUIT YOUR OPPONENT'S MOVEMENTS
070 -ENDURANCE:HOW TO OBTAIN MAXIMUM ENDURANCE
071 -THE DEADLY SIDEKICK-MASTER THE MOST POWERFUL KICK OF COMBAT
077 -JOINT-LOCKS:HOW TO CONTROL YOUR OPPONENT
087 -SUPER LEG CONDITIONING: ENDURANCE,STRENGTH,FLEXIBILITY, and AGILITY
088 -CONTROL KICKING: KICK 10 TIMES or MORE WITHOUT DROPPING YOUR FOOT TO THE GROUND
091 -HOW TO CLOSE THE GAP: COVERS FOOTWORK and DISTANCING
092 -THE ART OF EVASION: IF THEY CAN'T HIT YOU, THEY CAN'T BEAT YOU!!
093 -TELEGRAPHING: LEARN TO PREDICT YOUR OPPONENT'S MOVES!!

*OUR COMPANY PAYS FOR ALL THE SHIPPING, NO MATTER HOW MANY TAPES YOU BUY!! PLEASE SEND U.S. or Canadian Funds Only!! Order-Form Below:

TAPE #	QUANTITY	NAME OF VIDEO-TAPE	PRICE
			TOTAL

NAME:_____ ADDRESS:_____ CITY:_____
STATE/PROVINCE:_____ ZIP/POSTAL CODE:_____ PHONE: (___) ___-____

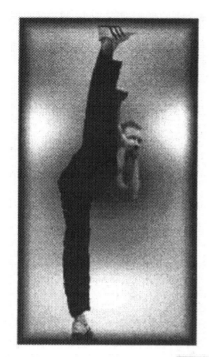

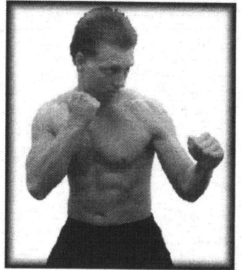

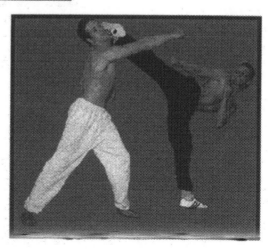

Printed in the United States
By Bookmasters